BREAK THROUGH
BINGE EATING

BREAK THROUGH
BINGE EATING

The Simple Solution to Ending Your Struggles with Food and Your Body

Beth Riley, MSW, LISW-CP, CEDS-S

Table of Contents

Introduction

In 23 years as a therapist, I've sat across from hundreds of people who have come to find relief from their struggles with food and their bodies.

Early on in my career, I began to develop a passion for working with women suffering from binge eating and other overeating behaviors. Most clients would show up to their first appointment in a state of desperation after years of being stuck in a vicious cycle of dieting and gaining the weight back. Once they discovered that I was not there to judge or criticize them and that there was a reason they were turning to food, most of them felt an immediate sense of relief and hope.

In the beginning years of my practice, many clients came to me directly from weight loss programs where they had become obsessed with counting points, carbs, or fat grams. They were frustrated each time they got on the scale and it didn't budge. Others came straight from their doctor's office after being told they were prediabetic, needed to lose weight and handed a sheet of paper with a diet to follow – as if they didn't already think they needed to shed a few pounds and hadn't been trying for years.

The health and wellness industry is booming with products and services claiming to increase your energy, prevent or reverse disease, and make you feel good about yourself. Enticing ads pop up on social media seducing you into thinking this is the one that will finally help you shed the unwanted weight, fit into your desired jean size, and find true happiness.

Going out to lunch with a group of women means a guaranteed conversation about the latest cleanse, fast, workout program or health regimen. The current buzz is plant-based dieting and intermittent fasting. I am not here to criticize any particular diet or lifestyle choice but to point out that for anyone prone to disordered eating, perfectionism, or taking things to extremes, some of these approaches can do more harm than good.

What is not being mentioned is that when no one is looking, many who are trying to live with rigid food rules end up sneaking into the kitchen after everyone else is in bed and stuffing themselves with all the foods they aren't supposed to eat. They are eating a salad for lunch in front of their friends and then making a beeline to the nearest drive-through for a burger and fries.

They are miserable and beating themselves up thinking everyone can do it but them. They think they are failures and berate themselves for not being able to stick to a diet. One client told me she had spent "tens of thousands of dollars on diets" yet felt a sense of "hopelessness."

Problems arise for some people when they follow extreme diets. Firstly, eliminating foods they enjoy can lead to feelings of deprivation and eventually to overeating these foods. Second, if they were turning to those foods for comfort or to manage stress, they are likely going to experience overwhelming emotions and increased stress when they can't eat cookies to numb themselves. If they don't return to overeating, they might seek relief in what I refer to as companion behaviors, like drinking, drugs, or excessive spending.

For most of my clients, the pattern is similar.

Sometimes it begins in childhood or early adolescence with someone telling you that you are fat and/or growing up in a family where weight, shape, and appearance are emphasized. One or both parents become concerned about their child's weight or maybe it's the child itself who's upset because they're being bullied at school or by their siblings. They see the pediatrician who notices the number on the scale has gone up significantly and then tells the family that the child needs to watch their weight.

This scenario typically takes place during prepuberty, when girls are actually supposed to gain 20–40 pounds in their midsection to prepare for menses. Some boys gain during this time too in preparation for a growth spurt. Panic sets in for the child and parents. The child thinks he or she is bad and there's something wrong with them. The doctor might recommend a diet and increased exercise. The family follows the doctor's advice, and the scene is set for a lifetime of poor body image, low self-esteem, disordered eating, or a full-blown eating disorder.

Many clients have shared with me that when they look at pictures from their youth, they were normal sized and wish they had seen that at the time.

Other clients go to college and gain weight their first year then end up in a vicious cycle of yo-yo dieting in a desperate attempt to shed the unwanted pounds. Still others gain a lot of weight during pregnancy, become distressed, and begin a pattern of restricting and overeating.

I've found that many of my clients start new diets when they have an event on the horizon – a wedding, college reunion, or a beach vacation.

See if this sounds familiar. You think to yourself that you have to lose 20 pounds before showing up to your family reunion at the beach. So, you decide to start the diet program you saw advertised on social media. You also join a gym. You stock the fridge with everything you are going to eat for the next week and then set out to meticulously follow the regimen. You indulge in one final binge before you begin.

You follow the plan exactly for a few days, maybe even a week or longer. Then you get busy. Let's say you have an out-of-town work conference or several social events in a row. You're stressed, exhausted, and feeling overwhelmed. You can't seem to fit the exercise into your schedule for a few days. There's tempting food everywhere.

You take that first bite of a cookie and the downward spiral begins. You immediately tell yourself you've blown it. One cookie becomes the entire box followed by other foods you've have been craving. You might be thinking "I'll start over tomorrow," but when tomorrow arrives, you are tired and stressed and beating yourself up for eating the forbidden foods. It's over and the cycle begins anew.

Many people alternate between eating only "healthy" food and pounding on a treadmill every morning or lying on the sofa eating junk food. They are either being "good" or "bad" and there's no in between. They feel out of control around certain foods and think the only way to avoid eating too much of the "bad" foods is to eliminate them completely, but that only lasts so long, and when they eat one of those foods again, they end up consuming even more than before.

They envy their friends, coworkers, or partners who they perceive as capable of sticking to a rigid regimen of eating "clean" and doing extreme workouts every day.

They feel stuck, even miserable, because their very existence is determined by how much they weigh and what size they wear.

By the time they reach my office or buy my book, they are sick and tired of living this way. They tell me I'm their last resort.

Their stories share common themes: "I'm not loveable," "I'm ugly," "I'm the fattest one in the room," or "there's something wrong with me."

Many of these people, particularly women, are able to maintain a pace and level of competence that is superhuman, yet they think they aren't doing enough.

I've counseled many teachers, nurses, and helping professionals over the years. They are great at taking care of others but tend to put themselves last on the list. Without realizing it, they have been turning to food to help cope with their stress.

These women are the supreme caretakers of the world.

I've worked with lawyers, doctors, and even high-powered executives who starved themselves, berated themselves, and worked themselves to the bone, never taking time off to rest. Some would head straight to a drive-through or grocery store on their way home and then sit in front of their TVs, numbing themselves from the day's stresses with as much sweet, salty, or crunchy food as they could eat. Others would drink a bottle or two of wine each night to achieve their desired state of numbness. Some would consume large quantities of food and wine.

All of these clients thought they were losing their minds until I explained they had figured out their own way to survive – that these behaviors were serving a purpose in their lives.

What makes "Break Through Binge Eating" different?

This book is going to help you get to the underlying reasons why you overeat and abuse your body. Unlike other books on overeating, I'll be addressing those "companion behaviors" too. You may notice that sometimes I refer to all these behaviors as "self-destructive" and other times I may use the word "self-preserving." The bottom line is that there is a reason you turn to them.

What I know from personal and professional experience is that if you simply focus on one of these behaviors, the others will rear their ugly heads over time. My intention is to empower you to overcome all of them. If you adopt the practices in this book, you won't need them anymore.

This is not a radical approach. It's based on what I refer to as developing the "moderation mindset." There's actually no right or wrong way. It's a path that evolves as you become more attuned to your authentic self and learn to treat yourself with kindness and compassion.

You are going to rediscover the real you – that child inside you who was born knowing what they wanted and needed until the world started telling you who you were and how you should act. You will learn to connect with your inner wisdom and strength that's been there all along.

How I decided to write this book

About a year ago, I finally realized that I was suffering from severe burnout. I am sure others saw it long before I did. So, I made the gut-wrenching decision to leave behind the eating disorder treatment center I had grown from scratch. I wasn't exactly sure what I wanted to do next which was scary.

I started doing what I do best which is networking and ended up visiting a wellness center not far from where I live.

The owners of this particular center are two enlightened women who recognized that many of their guests had problems with overeating and body image. Since working with binge eating is my area of specialty, they asked me to lead some retreats for their guests and to create a cutting-edge curriculum for them.

So, with a sense of excitement and fear – this was a completely new venture, after all – I made my way up the windy mountain roads to the retreat center for the first workshop. Fortunately, the route is surrounded by panoramic views of the Blue Ridge Mountains, and with each curve of the road, I could feel my angst subside as I took in the breathtaking vistas. I started feeling connected to my creative self and began to believe that everything was going to be OK. I was on the right path.

I spent the next three days alongside a group of incredible women. I sat with them through every meal and snack. At times, emotions came up as they let down their guard and expressed their real feelings. I felt honored to be there to support them and watch them heal.

At first the participants were reluctant to let go of the diet mentality and the idea that exercise had to be punishing to be effective. By the end of the week, they were able to eat foods they had been avoiding in moderation. They also learned to give themselves permission to sleep in occasionally or take a mindful walk in the woods instead of attending circuit training every morning.

I had tears in my eyes as I witnessed the transformation between not only their relationship with food but with themselves. They were opening up to each other, expressing their fears, anxieties, and hopes. It was more than I could have ever hoped for in a four-day workshop.

But I also noticed these women (and a couple of men who enrolled in the next few workshops) struggled with giving themselves permission to slow down. They were uncomfortable with unstructured time, not knowing how to just be still.

The results of the workshops were all I had hoped for and more. By the time they finished the week, most of the participants understood what had led to their overeating and other self-destructive behaviors and had stopped beating up on themselves. They recognized the importance of giving themselves time to rest. They became aware that stress reduction and increasing their connection with their authentic selves were the keys to healing.

The Healing Path

In today's increasingly complex society, we are desperately seeking relief from overwhelming stressors. We are trapped in a web of busyness that creates a state of what I refer to as "high freeze." We are completely disconnected from what we need to thrive as human beings. In this world of "human doing," we are too busy to help ourselves, so we reach for ways to avoid, escape, and numb.

There's a lot of information about health and wellness out there. Self-help books are being published at record rates and people are devouring them. There are huge, sold-out conferences promising the key to happiness and healing. Self-care is all the rage, yet we are more stressed out and miserable than ever. We live in an intense time, and our behaviors reflect it.

I am all too familiar with living in a frenzied state completely disconnected to myself and what I value. It wasn't until I left my corporate job over a year ago that I realized how deep into misery I had sunk. Fortunately, I hadn't turned to self-destructive behaviors, but that's only because I have a lot of good coping tools and support.

I am excited to share with you both my personal experience and the valuable tools and skills I have learned, taught my clients, and practiced myself over the years.

After reading this book, you will no longer obsess over every morsel you put in your mouth or whether you walked 10,000 steps in a day. You'll be more comfortable in your body and discover movement doesn't have to be punishing or painful.

With your newfound tools and changed attitude toward self-care, you will be liberated from the vicious cycle of dieting, overeating, feeling shame and hopelessness, and then dieting again. This punishing lifestyle is going to end for good, and without doing anything radical you will find freedom from the burdensome obsession of food, weight, and your body. You will finally be free to live a life that is not controlled by what you or others are eating or what size pants you wear.

My approach will help you:

- Learn to find a sense of peace with your body.
- Take a hard look at all the behaviors you turn to and learn the tools you need to eliminate them.
- Discover the joy that comes from living a life that is focused on what's really important to you rather than on changing or perfecting your body.
- Uncover your creative self/inner longings.
- Make room to deepen your connections with others and have more meaningful relationships.
- Learn to live in the "rainbow zone" between black and white and all or nothing.

What I am offering is a path to true healing from your disordered eating and other self-defeating behaviors. I have witnessed hundreds of women (and some men too) use this model and go on to live meaningful lives free of food, body, and weight obsession.

It works. All you have to do is be willing to take the leap. I promise the safety net is there.

Eating disorders, disordered eating, and "normal eating"

What's the difference between disordered eating and an eating disorder?

Disordered eating refers to a range of abnormal behaviors related to food consumption – eating to cope with stress, for instance, or binge eating – and shares some characteristics with full-blown eating disorders. An eating disorder is a serious and potentially life-threatening medical and mental illness that warrants treatment by specialists.

A disordered eater may restrict their food intake one day and then binge that night, but they only do it once a month. The difference between these behaviors and a full-blown eating disorder is generally the level of severity and the frequency of the behaviors. If you want more information about eating disorder diagnoses, go to **www.nationaleatingdisorders.org**.

Another term you may have heard is "normal eating." This refers to someone who eats regularly, is open to eating most foods, may not eat enough, or eats a little too much at times, mostly because of what's available or what's going on in their lives at that moment. A normal eater does not spend time stressing about what they just ate or will be eating later. Their lives do not revolve around their food choices or eating behaviors.

Disordered eating is often accompanied by those companion behaviors – all of which indicate that your life is off-kilter. As you heal your relationship with food and your body, the rest of your life will begin to fall into place. Ultimately, this book is meant to transform how you live your life.

The steps for ending your obsession with food, weight, and your body:

- End dieting. It's self-punishment, stressful, and unhealthy.
- Develop a realistic and sustainable approach to eating and exercise.
- Increase awareness of emotions, body sensations, and thoughts that could be triggering overeating or other self-destructive behaviors.
- Reduce your stress level and learn real self-care.
- Treat yourself with more kindness and compassion.
- Align your life with your values, those things that give your life meaning and joy.
- Learn to eat what you enjoy in moderation without overeating or guild—yes, even chocolate cake and ice cream.
- Develop a plan for staying on course no matter what life sends your way.

Intuitive eating, mindful eating and structured eating are some of the approaches you may have heard about or even tried.

Intuitive eating is allowing yourself to have what your body wants when it feels right. It's essentially tuning to your body's wisdom to make choices about food that feel good to you and your body.

Mindful eating means paying attention to your food along with any thoughts, feelings, or bodily sensations that occur while you are eating.

My personal experience, training, and years of counseling have led me to the conclusion that structured eating is typically the best place to start.

There are many reasons to begin with a regular eating pattern – the main one being that most disordered eaters have an inconsistent, even chaotic eating style and simply adding regularity to their meals and snacks reduces their stress.

I also suggest that along with establishing a structured eating plan, it is helpful to begin learning how to eat mindfully. I will provide suggestions about mindful eating in Chapter 11.

Preparing for your journey

If you are reading this, you are probably a woman in her 30s or older who may be struggling with more than one disordered behavior as a way to cope with unresolved life issues or stress. You could be burned out from work or from taking care of everyone around you while making it seem like you have it all together. You don't take time for yourself and probably think that it is selfish or wasteful to do so. You are at the end of your rope but may not even have realized it until now.

If you are younger than 30, male or LGBTQ, I want you to know that I have you in mind, too. Disordered eating does not discriminate.

Before I launch into my story, I suggest that you either purchase a journal or find one that's been lying around waiting to have a purpose. If you don't have one handy, just use a legal pad or scrap paper for now. For those of you who prefer using an electronic device, I ask that you consider going the old-fashioned route and put pen to paper. I want you to use the journal to jot down a quick thought or doodle or to scribble emotions as they arise.

You'll find a number of activities in this book that will challenge you to reflect, observe, and reach – exercises that are designed to help you get to the core of why you turn to overeating and other unhealthy behaviors and to introduce you to opportunities to stretch and grow. This is where your journal can come in handy. Remember, this is not a class and there is no test at the end. You can read the book without doing any of the activities, you can pick and choose, or you can come back to them when you feel up to it. It's your journey, so choose a pace you are comfortable with.

It would be helpful to start thinking about a "safe person" or two in your life – a friend or family member you can confide in as you take this journey – someone who won't judge and who will support you and will help hold you accountable.

This book is not meant to replace therapy or medical treatment. If you are currently seeing a mental health or medical professional for treatment of an eating disorder, disordered eating, or any other issue, please don't discontinue with them. Inform your providers that you are reading this book and perhaps suggest they read it, too, so they can learn about this approach and be supportive as you take this journey.

It is not unusual for those who suffer from overeating behaviors to also have mental health issues. Many of my clients have been diagnosed with depression, anxiety, or mood disorders.

If you have a mental health diagnosis and are reading this book, I recommend that you inform your loved ones and/or mental health provider that you are working on changing your eating behaviors. As you reduce or eliminate those behaviors that have helped you avoid the underlying reasons for escape, you might become overwhelmed by emotions

If you have suicidal thoughts or urges to self-harm at any time while reading this book, tell your loved one or support person immediately. If you are alone, call 911, the National Suicide Hotline at 800-273-8255, or your local crisis line.

For those of you who don't have a mental health diagnosis, I recommend that you stay alert to any increase in emotions like sadness or anxiety or changes in behavior that may indicate you need more support. If you experience any thoughts of suicide or self-harm, please reach out to the above resources. I intentionally provide coping tools throughout this book, but it's good to be prepared just in case.

As with any journey worth taking, there are potential hazards along the way. Awareness and preparation are the best tools for ensuring you arrive safely at your destination.

About me

My name is Beth Riley. I am a certified eating disorder specialist, and I have dedicated my life to helping those suffering from eating and body image issues.

I've devoted more than two decades to learning about, treating and training others to understand this complex mental illness and related issues. I've been fortunate to have worked alongside and studied under some of the leading experts in the fields of overeating, obesity, fitness, and nutrition, and I felt it was my duty and a privilege to pass on their knowledge along with what I've learned from my work and my personal experience.

I have trained therapists, dietitians, coaches, and teachers. I've also spent a lot of time educating doctors and other healthcare providers, since most medical schools don't cover eating disorders, instead focusing primarily on obesity prevention.

I am constantly pursuing knowledge about advances in the fields of eating disorders, nutrition, and mental health and wellness. When I'm not speaking at a professional conference, I'm sitting in my seat taking notes. Yes, I'm a quintessential nerd.

I've owned, operated, and sold a successful eating disorder treatment center. I'm also a speaker, educator, and mentor to many women in our field.

I had fantasized about being an author since childhood, but as the years went by that vision was displaced by the reality of having to provide for my family and my insecurity that I did not have anything to offer. I told myself that I wasn't qualified, that I didn't have the skills to write a book, that I was too busy. Fortunately, taking a yearlong sabbatical from working in an office setting granted me the opportunity to find some creative space for myself. So, I started writing, and with a lot of encouragement from friends, loved ones, and colleagues, I realized my dream. It feels good.

My story

My father's family was obsessed with weight and appearances. It was probably related to the fact that the family owned a woman's clothing company started by great grandfather. I grew up surrounded by models, photographers, and fashion designers.

Since the business was located in New York City and had factories in South Carolina, I split my childhood residences between the two which meant I never quite felt like I belonged in either place.

After attending elementary school in South Carolina where I was a star student, I ended up in an all-female private school in Manhattan in a classroom full of brilliant and talented girls. I felt lost and of course inadequate from the start.

Starting around this time, I began to restrict my food. My diet consisted of no breakfast, a small container of coffee-flavored yogurt, and a green apple for lunch and dinner with my parents if they were around – if they weren't, I wouldn't eat. I remember going to bed with a gnawing feeling in my stomach and a sense of accomplishment.

In hindsight, it was inevitable that I would develop a disordered relationship with food and my body.

At the end of my 10th grade year, I decided to attend boarding school since my brother had plans to attend one the coming fall, and I didn't want to be left at home alone.

I had a lot of social anxiety and fear of eating in front of other people. Also, I was worried about gaining weight by eating "unhealthy" cafeteria food. So, I mostly ate grapefruit and tuna out a can in my dorm room.

Then I discovered that a girl across the hall from me had lots of food in her room – all the "unhealthy" junk I craved but never allowed myself to eat – like popcorn, cookies, ice cream, and chips.

She would invite me over late at night to share these forbidden foods. I started with a little popcorn. It turned into a lot of popcorn. Then came the ice cream – lots of ice cream. I would eat so much that I would be in pain and not be able to sleep. I couldn't seem to get enough.

Of course, I gained a lot of weight and was horrified at the thought of anyone at home seeing me in this larger body. When I look back at it now, I realize that I was experiencing shame.

Drinking became another way for me to relieve my anxiety and help me let go and have fun. My low self-esteem made me socially awkward, but when I drank my inhibitions disappeared and I became the life of the party.

The food and alcohol were my attempts to cope with stress and low self-worth. I honestly don't know how I functioned but somehow, I did. I even managed to get good grades.

For college, I set my sights high and ended up at Stanford University surrounded by overachievers and perfectionists. In an attempt to cope with the stress of moving across country and starting over again, I began a restrictive diet and exercise regimen a few months before I left for California.

When I arrived in my all freshman dorm of 400, I immediately felt out of place and overwhelmed. I managed my feelings by establishing a rigid routine of restricting and intense exercise that I maintained the first two years there.

I decided to spend my junior year in Italy. I ended up renting an apartment on the outskirts of Florence by myself. I thought I would be okay living alone, but I ended up feeling isolated and depressed.

This time instead of starving myself, I turned to food for comfort and wine to drown out my loneliness. I gained a lot of weight but didn't care until I started thinking about returning home. I began to panic so went on a rigid diet. I could not let anyone at home see that I had gained weight. It was shame again.

By the time I arrived home, I had done it – all the weight I had gained was gone and then some. The first thing my father said when he saw me was how thin I looked and how glad he was I hadn't gained weight. Success.

Beyond college

After college, I stayed in San Francisco but struggled finding a good job. I was depressed. I remember going to a holistic doctor who told me that all my problems were related to an overabundance of yeast in my body. So, I started what would become a two-year fast/cleanse that eliminated all bread, dairy, and sugar – even fruit.

It was when I moved to North Carolina at age 24 that things really went downhill.

I had accepted a job as director of a nonprofit in a small town near Asheville. It was a high stress job that involved a lot of social events and being in the media.

I stayed on the restrictive diet I brought with me from California, but it didn't last long. After a few months, I began a new cycle of bingeing.

For the next two years, I would go home after work and gorge on ice cream, cookies, and chips. Because I was horrified of gaining weight and everyone in the small community noticing, I was desperate to find a way to get rid of the food.

Within months I was living in my own personal hell and had started to get rid of my binges by vomiting.

What started as an occasional release became a daily habit.

By the time I was 27, I was sick and tired of self-destructing. I reached out to a friend and told her my dark secret. She encouraged me to seek professional help so I checked myself into a center. I was ready.

When I was in treatment, I remember marveling at one of the therapists as she demonstrated that she could eat a handful of M&Ms without consuming the entire bag. I was certain that would never happen to me, but it did – not immediately – but gradually over the course of the next few years.

For many years now, I have lived in a place of moderation – what I call the "rainbow zone" with food and exercise. I am still a work in progress related to my issue with perfectionism and overachieving, but I no longer turn to substances to cope. I'm better at slowing down and paying attention to my need to rest and restore.

I'm a big believer in the healing power of nature and animals and find peace in simple acts like watching the birds at the feeder in my yard or snuggling with my rescue dogs Jasper and Joni.

SECTION 1:
What is this stuff we are doing?

CHAPTER 1: Taking stock of our lives

When it comes to pursuing happiness, we can be our own worst enemy.

We're stressed. We're always "on." We have external pressure to push ourselves past our limits, and we put even more pressure on ourselves on top of that. Then we put our bodies through the wringer trying to make them look perfect.

The relentless quest for body perfection

Our poor bodies. They are never good enough. We are surrounded by women who have flawless, wrinkle-free skin, sparkling white teeth, and perfectly sculpted bodies. It's rare to find a woman in her natural state. When we look back at photos of middle-aged women from our grandmothers' era, we see gray hair, wrinkles, and flabby bodies. It was the norm. Now, it's hard to discern a mother from her adult daughter.

Jane Fonda is a perfect example. She certainly does not look like anyone's grandmother. It strikes me as odd that mothers and grandmothers today often look more it, have whiter teeth and better skin than their daughters. It's no wonder teenage girls and women in their 20s are getting veneers, chin implants, breast augmentations or reductions, liposuction, or a number of other cosmetic procedures. They are in a race to keep up with the older generation.

Acne is like a death sentence now. Those who can afford it see a dermatologist and take medicine as soon as they get their first pimple. Our children have zero tolerance for any flaws on their body. It's no one's fault. We are being constantly exposed to body perfection.

As we age, there's a lot of pressure to look younger which is not necessarily a bad thing. It's when the pursuit of a youthful appearance or perfect body results in undue stress or is misaligned with our values, it can be problematic. If you feel compelled to buy more and more products, have multiple surgeries to change your appearance, or consistently can't take a day off from the gym to have fun with your friends, then you have likely crossed into unhealthy territory.

I am not judging or faulting you. An entire industry has developed for the sole purpose of convincing us that we need to be all these things to be happy.

We are expected to look perfect at every stage of life. Photos are plastered across social media starting with mom's first ultrasound. The onslaught of photos of ourselves on social media creates a lot of internalized pressure to look your best at all times – during puberty, during pregnancy, and even immediately after childbirth (think Kate Middleton).

Women are supposed to be thin, toned, wrinkle free, and youthful. Older men can have gray hair and wrinkles, but there's an unspoken rule that gray hair and facial lines are taboo for women. We have also been encouraged to hide our fat and curves so many women squeeze themselves into super tight and seriously uncomfortable underwear.

Fortunately, some companies and women are changing the dialogue with more focus on real body sizes and shapes. Still, dressing rooms in women's clothing stores can be dark places. Try standing in one and you're likely to hear comments like "my thighs look enormous", "you can wear that because you're thin, but I wouldn't dare," or "if I lost about 30 pounds, these pants would look a lot better on me."

Most of us have something negative to say about certain parts of our bodies, especially as we stand in front of the mirror getting dressed in the morning. Judging ourselves and others based on size and appearance has become the norm, and it's such a tragic waste of time and energy. It drains our joy.

What is the last thing you said to your body? Did you, for instance, tell yourself you couldn't wear a specific pair of jeans because your thighs looked too big?

We are constantly yelling at our bodies, calling them names we wouldn't dare use on anyone else. I often ask my clients what they think their lives would be like if they couldn't see their bodies or anyone else's. What about if the ideal body type was curvy and a larger size?

As long as we focus on our bodies and what we perceive to be wrong with them, we don't have as much space in our heads to devote to what's really going on with us – and certainly no room for pursuing joy. It's much easier to fixate on our outer selves, our cellulite, or the wrinkles on our forehead than acknowledge that we are lonely or dissatisfied with our lives.

I was shocked when I was shopping with my daughter (now in college) at a vintage clothing store in New Orleans recently, and there were two women celebrating their hips and butts. They would come out of the dressing room, look at themselves in the mirror, twirl around to see their bodies from every angle, and shout, "I look so hot in this dress!" It sent shivers down my spine to hear women being not just kind to their bodies, but truly admiring them.

What our children are learning

The desperation to be thin and sculpted often starts in childhood. I've worked with girls as young as 8 who are counting their steps, measuring the girth of their midsections, and weighing themselves every morning.

I will never forget when my daughter was in first grade and said, "My tummy is big, Mommy." I was horrified. She certainly had not heard those words from me. At the time, she had been playing with a girl whose mother constantly made negative comments about her weight and body. I couldn't fault the mother – it was all she knew to do.

The war on our bodies starts early, and the battlefield is covered with landmines.

By age 6, girls especially start to express concerns about their weight or shape. Between 40 percent and 60 percent of elementary school girls (ages 6–12) are worried about their weight and becoming fat.[1] How could they not be? Everywhere they turn they are exposed to the message that thin is better.

It's not just girls and women who are on the ultimate quest for perfection, but boys and men, too. Starting at a very young age, boys are exposed to societal messages that they should be bulked up, lean, and have six-pack abs. Have you seen the muscles on action heroes, athletes, and celebrities these days? Their idols look like they've been working out eight hours a day, which they probably have.

Of American elementary school girls who read magazines, 69 percent say the pictures influence their concept of the ideal body shape. Nearly half (47 percent) say the pictures make them want to lose weight.[2] Children of mothers who are overly concerned about their weight are at increased risk for modeling those unhealthy attitudes and behaviors.[3] Nearly a third of children age 5 to 6 choose an ideal body size that is thinner than their current size.[4]

By age 6, children are aware of dieting and may have tried it.[5][6][7] Just over a quarter (26 percent) of 5-year-olds recommend dieting – not eating junk food, eating less overall – for someone who has gained weight, and roughly one in four children have tried some form of dieting by the time they are 7 years old.[7]

The trend continues as they grow older. From 2013 to 2016, almost 38 percent of American youth age 16 to 19 said they had tried to lose weight during the past year, according to the U.S. Centers for Disease Control and Prevention. A decade ago, that number was about 25 percent.

As you might expect, more girls than boys reported trying to lose weight (45 percent versus 30 percent). Hispanic teenagers of both genders reported weight loss attempts at higher rates than white, black, and Asian youth.

What makes these statistics alarming is that weight loss attempts outpaced the increase in childhood obesity rates, according to the CDC. Obesity rates among adolescents age 12 to 19 increased from 18.4 percent to almost 21 percent between 2009-2010 and 2015-2016. So, despite attempts to reduce weight bias and stigma, our young people still feel the need to reduce their body size in an attempt to it in with the thin ideal.

The problem with this hyper focus on weight, nutrition, and fitness is that it can increase stress levels, anxiety, and feelings of shame for those who are in the overweight or obese category or even normal weight people who worry they are or could be too heavy.

It can also contribute to disordered eating or even trigger full-blown eating disorders in people with a tendency to develop them. The most startling eating disorder statistic relates to children under age 12 – while hospitalizations involving eating disorders increased for all age groups in the decade ending in

2009, the number of hospitalizations for children under 12 surged 72 percent in that timeframe.[8]

Schools, doctors, and parents are on high alert to prevent obesity, with weigh-ins and BMI checks starting in elementary school. I've had a number of parents tell me their child came home from school feeling humiliated after being weighed in front of others in gym class, and that's when they began hiding food and bingeing.

Instead of being taught moderation, society is setting up children at early ages to think they have done something horribly wrong if they eat a cookie, and of course, these children become adults who end up seeing food the same way.

Programs in schools are teaching about "good foods" and "bad foods" starting at very young ages. The "good foods" are typically vegetables, low-fat proteins, whole grains, low-fat dairy, and fruit, while the "bad foods" are all those things they enjoy, such as cookies, ice cream, chips, fried foods, and sugary drinks. While we can agree the foods in the first group are healthier, the foods in the second are what kids generally love.

When you tell children that the foods they love are "bad," it creates the ideal setup for overeating those foods and/or eating those foods in secret and feeling guilt or shame when they do. For kids who are prone to developing eating disorders, this type of food labeling can lead to a full-blown illness.

Without realizing it, society is asking children to put a lot of thought into every bite of food which is causing stress on their young brains. If you are a parent, it's not your fault. You've been doing your best to navigate a complicated situation. Reading this book means you are now part of the solution.

There's a lot of confusing information out there. On the one hand, the medical community has led the charge on fixing our obesity problem. They cite evidence that obesity itself causes diseases such as cancer, diabetes, and heart disease. Others argue that obesity is not a disease and that we should love our bodies just as they are.

This is a complicated issue that is creating major divides in how we treat those with eating, weight, and body-related issues. It's become a literal minefield with each side throwing darts at the other. The true victim is the individual struggling to figure out what approach they need to take to feel better. I argue that individual choice is lacking on both sides and that most people inherently know what is best for them given the chance to explore their options.

For a child who happens to be born into a larger body, have a more muscular build or develop early, it's a minefield. In the current climate of "the thin ideal," these children are practically guaranteed a lifetime of body hatred, low self-worth, and shame.

Please try not to judge yourself for how you've been handling food with your children to this point. There's a lot of confusing information out there. I like to tell my clients "now you're in the solution."

I'm not suggesting you go out and stock your cabinets with junk food or to abandon all your healthy habits but instead to be aware of the potential negative impact of giving any food too much power.

My perspective is based on the premise that it is practically impossible to avoid consuming the "bad foods" without eventually overeating them. I want to empower you to be able to consume these foods in moderation without beating yourself up or feeling shame. If you discover that you are turning to certain foods to relieve stress or cope with unresolved emotions, this book will provide you with alternatives to help you feel better.

Measuring everything but our stress level

How many mornings do you wake up and the first thing you do is go to your bathroom and step on the scale? For some people, this may not make or break their day, but for many that number directly impacts their mood.

Not only can we measure our weight, body composition, steps, calories consumed and expended, heart rate, and more just by wearing a device on our arms or using an app – there are 318,000 health apps now and 340,000 wearable apps[9] – but we can easily compare our stats to what others are doing without even having to ask.

While these devices can serve as motivation for some people, they can trigger unhealthy behaviors – even obsession – in others. Research also suggests these measurement tools may encourage appearance-driven exercise over working out for purely health reasons.[10]

In the "wrong brain," I use this term when referring to those with obsessive or perfectionistic tendencies; it by no means suggests there is anything wrong with your brain, just that you are genetically predisposed to going to extremes – measuring can be disastrous. It can lead to a hyper focus on numbers and the thought that you are never doing enough.

The potential problem with focusing on numbers:

- You could become overly reliant on a standardized number and external source, causing you to not listen to your body's own cues. For example, you are sick or injured and exercise anyway since you feel compelled to meet your number goal for the day.
- The standards we are using to measure are not all based on evidence and facts, and they are constantly changing –

10,000 steps a day is an example of a measure that is not backed by science.

- Focusing on numbers may act as a motivator for some but can lead to obsession in others. Even worse, it can negatively impact your mood and lead to depression, anxiety, hopelessness, or low self-esteem.

Trying to feel our best

Almost every time we go on the internet, we're bombarded with ads for products that claim to help us cleanse toxins from our system, boost our energy, live longer, prevent aging, eliminate fat and cellulite, and of course lose weight.

I was raised in a culture of open-mindedness when it comes to natural remedies and supplements, and living in the San Francisco Bay Area in the 1980s only reinforced that view. I try to stay current on the best supplements and vitamins and believe some of them are beneficial.

We all deserve to feel good. The problem arises when we take it to the extreme. When our attempt at being healthy or living longer becomes obsessive or stressful or creates an imbalance in our lives.

Another issue is if we are turning to these products to solve problems that are related to stress, unresolved emotions, or dissatisfaction with our lives.

What if the reason you aren't sleeping is that you're up late at night trying to finish a work project that you could have delegated to someone else? Instead of looking to a supplement to boost your energy or get a better night's sleep, we're going to explore what I refer to as "real self-care."

I'm not suggesting you stop buying products or services that are helping you. I want you to simply get curious about the reasons you are choosing to use them and see if there are any other options that might heal you from the inside and produce lasting effects.

Living in "high freeze"

I use the term "high freeze" to describe our lives. Another phrase I like is "at the altar of busy." It seems that society's mantra is "the busier the better" and that our calendars should be packed full of activities.

Always busy. At home. In our car. In the airport. I remember how proud of myself I was when I figured out how to download Zoom, a virtual meeting app, on my iPhone. Little did I realize that would mean I could meet with anyone, anytime, and my down time would be sucked away.

I had a client who was an executive at a tech company. She was so immersed in work that she would forget to take breaks the entire day. (I know many of you can relate.) After some time in therapy, she began to realize that the stress of her relentless work pace was slowly killer her. She identified a need to rest and spend time enjoying nature as essential to her well-being. She decided to take a small step toward change by incorporating two 15-minute breaks in her day. She put them on her calendar with alerts. She would either go outside for a mindful walk around the parking lot without her phone, sip a cup of tea, or shut her office door and do a few yoga stretches or a guided meditation. These few, simple steps were life changing for her.

Thanks to smartphones, we are always plugged in. We are always "on," and we are getting more and more comfortable abandoning simple face-to-face conversations.

I've decided to make a practice of carving out some of my time in airports, on planes, or in waiting rooms to simply chill. I've discovered the art of staring out the window at the clouds or trees, noticing the art on the walls or simply closing my eyes and taking a few deep breaths.

Studies show that all work all the time is simply not as productive as we think. It puts us in a constant state of stress that is unhealthy.

One reason we find ourselves so busy is because we are constantly confronted with options. I had a friend in high school who referred to it as a "neuroses of options." Venture capitalist and author Patrick McGinnis coined the term FOBO – Fear of a Better Option – to describe the paralysis brought on by having so many options that it becomes difficult, if not impossible, to just make a decision.

As you progress on this journey, it is my hope that you'll learn to step back from the altar of busy, to understand the beauty of taking a few deep breaths, and to discover the art of staring out the window.

Caretakers of the world

For most of my life, I suffered from thinking I had to take responsibility for everything.

It was no surprise that in my marriage I put myself in the position to be the main breadwinner, the supermom, the resident doctor, the bookkeeper and tax preparer, the animal caretaker, and the chef. I often hear from my clients phrases like "It won't get done if I don't take care of it" or "It's easier if I just do it myself."

We wake up one day and realize this attitude has made us bitter, angry, and even resentful, not to mention miserable. We have carried the burden for so long that we don't even know how to ask for help. We conjure up in our minds that other women are capable of doing it all and that we must be weak or deeply flawed if we can't do as much as they do.

If we are completely self-reliant, we don't have to feel vulnerable. An important part of the journey to healing your relationship with food and your body is learning to let go of the need to do it all yourself. The process starts with noticing what it is you do that you could possibly turn over to someone else, either at work, home, or among your friends. It will probably mean that you are going to need to ask for help which can be uncomfortable at first, but once you get the hang of it, you'll wonder why it took you so long.

Ideally, the act of asking for help will not only lower your stress level, but also create more satisfying relationships that feel more like partnerships. It will also free up time for yourself to rest or even have some fun.

I didn't recognize how lopsided many of my relationships were until my husband and daughter pointed out that I was constantly on the phone trying to help someone. What I hadn't realized is that I was always giving and rarely asking for support for myself which was a recipe for burnout.

I do enjoy networking, connecting people, and helping others get started on their career paths, so I doubt I'll stop, but I am trying to be more selective so I can save time for rest and fun.

Can you think of areas in your life where you may be offering too much?

Dig deep. It took me a long time to figure out how much all of the giving was sucking the life out of me.

Staying in unhealthy job situations

Most of the time we find ways to justify staying in a job that's making us miserable. Of course, there are times when circumstances dictate that we can't leave even if we know we need to, but often we make excuses and say things to ourselves like "I'm not a quitter," "It must be me," "I can't leave my colleagues," or "Maybe it's not as bad as I think it is."

We have become so accustomed to working 24/7 that we have little idea of what's "normal" anymore. Many employers automatically expect us to answer our phones or respond to emails at night, during the weekends, and in some cases while on vacation. This creates chronic stress for employees, along with high levels of job dissatisfaction and burnout.

Companies have been attempting to address the problem through workplace health initiatives that focus on work-life balance and self-care. They offer free gym memberships and EAPs (Employee Assistance Programs), yet the unspoken rule is that they you need to be available 24/7.

The problem is that if we do take time for ourselves, we end up feeling guilty. I know a lot of people who refuse to stay home when they're sick because they worry, they will get behind with work.

I thought it was outrageous that Italians shut most everything down from noon to 3 p.m. when I lived there. They would go home, eat lunch at a table with their families, and maybe even take a nap before returning to work. I found it very inconvenient and thought they were just being lazy and decadent. Needless to say, my perspective has changed.

Technology fever

Part of the reason work stress can so easily take over our lives is because we all carry supercomputers in our pockets or purses or just have them lying around the house – and they connect us to everyone, all the time.

We have become a society that is more focused on a screen than the people or environment around us. It's rare to be in any public setting these days where our eyes are on each other, and if we want an ego boost, all we have to do is post on social media and wait for the likes and emojis to pop up.

Granted, there is a lot of good that comes with technology. You can find many apps for mindfulness, for example, or improving your mental health. I am a big fan of online-guided meditations and instructional yoga videos.

With practice, you can learn how to live in the rainbow zone with technology.

"I'm not good enough"

This is the mantra of every woman I've ever had the privilege of sitting across from in my office: "I'm not good enough." Many of the women came from dysfunctional family systems but even those that didn't wound up thinking this way for various reasons.

My "I'm not good enough" message is what I internalized from my childhood. My parents were both extroverts and expected me to want to be more social. I constantly felt like I was disappointing them when I complained about all the extracurricular activities they had me do.

Then I married a man who constantly put pressure on me to be more social (thankfully, once he became a high school teacher that ended). Instead of being more compassionate toward myself, I ended up trying to please him by doing everything he wanted. You see I thought it was me – that I was the problem. It took years for me to realize that I had a right to want to rest when I got home.

Now I stop myself and ask if I really want to do something. That doesn't mean that at times I'm not going to make sacrifices or compromises for others, but I'm committed to speaking my voice and giving myself permission to say no.

There are so many ways to think you're not good enough: as a friend, colleague, spouse or partner, mother, daughter, relative, and even neighbor. I've counseled women who are literally driving themselves into frenzies trying to be everything to everyone.

These same women are constantly trying to prove themselves by doing more, taking on added responsibilities to try to find relief their negative thoughts and from overwhelming feelings of emptiness.

It's a vicious cycle that leads to a sense of powerlessness and ultimately to a dependence on self-destructive aka self-preserving behaviors to find relief. One effect of thinking you're not good enough is squelching your voice, holding in your true feelings and thoughts. It makes sense if you don't think you are worthy of being heard. Unfortunately, repressing your voice is a major trigger to overeating and those other self-defeating behaviors. It's like trying to keep a lid on a boiling pot of water.

Can you relate to thinking you are not good enough? Where did you get the message that you weren't enough? Where did you find the evidence for this? Or was it based on someone else's version of what it means to be enough?

Shoulding *yourself*

I have an endless and repeating list of shoulds: I should be a better mother, daughter, sister, aunt, friend. I should have people over to our house more often. I should do weight training to keep my bones healthy.

Most of my clients have their own long lists of shoulds. Can you relate to any of these?

- "I should be getting up at 5 and going to the gym."
- "I should have a perfectly clean and neat home."

- "I should eat healthier."
- "I should be further along in my life and my career."
- "I should be happy."
- "I should be thinner."

Shoulding may help some people to accomplish their goals. The problem is that over time it erodes our sense of self-worth and ultimately backfires as a method of sustaining our motivation over the long term.

It's like facing a demanding boss with unrealistic expectations, only that boss is inside our own heads. We have become accustomed to listening to the harsh voice that tells us we need to always be doing better. It's like yelling at yourself. It's exhausting and draining and ultimately counterproductive. We don't even realize how miserable we are making ourselves.

Reflect:

What are your shoulds? Write them down and then say them aloud to yourself.

Observe:

Notice how harsh they are. Ask yourself what purpose they have served in your life. Have they helped you keep functioning at a high level? Are they a way to stay connected to your parents or other important people from your childhood?

Reach:

Try naming that voice in your head. I call mine the "bitchy boss."

When I notice I'm shoulding myself or yelling at myself, I say to myself, "I hear you, bitchy boss, but I choose not to pay attention to what you are telling me to do."

Next time you hear the "should voice" or have a self-defeating thought, use this new approach: acknowledge the voice, refer to it by its name (i.e., the bitchy boss), and tell it that you hear it. Repeat its name and what it's saying to you in your head or out loud. You can even acknowledge that it makes sense you have this voice in your head. Then tell it you are choosing not to listen to it at this time. When it returns, repeat this process. The voice may not ever go away, but you can learn to handle it differently so that it doesn't have as much power over your mood or behaviors.

Who says you don't deserve it?

We think others can succeed but not us. We think others can have love, happiness, fulfillment, or financial success but that we are not smart enough, thin enough, or whatever else we can come up with that means we don't deserve these things.

I counseled a highly successful woman who was convinced she didn't deserve to be loved. Her father had abandoned her family when she was a child. Her interpretation of why he left was that she was too fat. After her father left, she started bingeing on sweets in her room and then began dieting and bingeing as a teenager. Years later, when her husband left her, she came to the same conclusion that it was due to her weight. The diet/binge cycle continued until in her mid-40s she started therapy.

After recognizing the underlying reasons for her lack of self-worth and learning alternate ways to cope other than bingeing, she was able to move forward with her life. She realized she didn't need a man to validate her and that she could find satisfaction in knowing she was OK on her own. Eventually she did marry a man who treated her with respect and was supportive.

Her story isn't unique.

Many of my clients have come to believe they do not deserve good things to happen to them. Often this mentality stems from their childhood or adverse life experiences. In some cases, their faulty belief system leads them to stop trying when they get close to success or even to sabotage themselves when they finally reach their goals.

This past year and a half has been a challenge for me since I made the decision to leave my corporate job and the big paycheck that went with it. It was a huge risk and has been a struggle financially for me and my family.

Without even realizing it, I fell back into my old mindset of thinking I wasn't good enough.

Fortunately, I had already started seeing a business coach (Gail) who is also a therapist who helped convince me this was old and faulty thinking. I also reached out to my colleagues for support, and they reminded me that I had succeeded before and could do it again. At times it felt as if they believed in me more than I did.

Steven Covey coined the term "abundance mentality" or "abundance mindset" in his 1989 bestseller The 7 Habits of Highly Effective People. He defined this as "a concept in which a person believes there are enough resources and successes to share with others." The opposite of the abundance mindset is the "scarcity mindset," which is based on the idea that if someone else is successful, then you can't be, too.[11]

Since Covey's book, the abundance mindset has become widely recognized as an integral component of overall well-being in the realm of personal and spiritual development.

It is likely that the only person telling you don't deserve good things in your life is you. It is my hope that in reading this book, you will recognize your self-defeating messages, learn to talk back to them, and ultimately believe that you deserve abundance in your life.

CHAPTER 2:
Trying to escape our problems

Running. Running from everything. Running away from issues with our partner, boss, job, friends. Instead of facing our problems, we try to find ways to avoid or delay dealing with them. It's so tempting to want to escape, especially when we know it's going to take a lot of energy and might bring up emotions we don't want to face.

Some methods of escape may be more obvious than others – overeating, for instance, or consistent or excessive use of alcohol or drugs – but running from our problems can come in so many other forms: overworking, excessive shopping, over focus on our children, and even obsessing about our weight, appearance, or health. The litmus test for determining if you are avoiding is having that nagging feeling inside that something isn't right.

Using food to cope

Overeating is an easy way to self-medicate. You can find food anywhere and now any time, thanks to developments like Uber Eats, 24-hour drive-throughs, and convenience stores on every corner. As this book was being prepared for publication, Forbes reported that Uber Eats was beginning to test food deliveries via drone in San Diego – the first test deliveries were from a McDonald's.

Food can help manage your emotions even when you are not aware you are experiencing them. In fact, food can help you avoid your emotions altogether.

If you're stressed out at work and doughnuts are in the staff kitchen, those soft, sugary treats can be comforting. If you spend the day rushing around town taking your kids from one place to the next, the fast food you eat in the car on the way to the next activity is like a drug. If you had a fight with your partner after dinner, that pint of ice cream you eat after they go to bed can help temporarily soothe you. If you live alone and feel a sense of emptiness in the evenings, then sitting in front of the TV with a box of your favorite cookies is a form of companionship.

When food isn't enough: adding alcohol and other substances to the mix

Many people I've counseled over the years engage in more than one self-destructive behavior (i.e., overeating and drinking). I've met many high-powered professionals who have extremely disordered eating, consume several drinks a day, and still function at a high level. They might not even realize they are being self-destructive, because those behaviors are so normalized in our society – everyone around them is doing the same.

If you are drinking more than you intend or feel your alcohol or drug use is out of control, this could be a sign of a substance use disorder. If that is the case, I suggest you consult a professional with experience treating addictions.

The substances most frequently abused by people with disordered eating or full-blown eating disorders include caffeine, tobacco, alcohol, laxatives, emetics, diuretics, appetite suppressants (such as amphetamines), heroin, and cocaine.[12] Roughly 20 percent of men and women being treated for substance use disorders reported binge eating.[13]

For those of you who have not been diagnosed with a substance use disorder but feel compelled to find relief from your everyday life by turning to drinking or a recreational drug, I encourage you to consider what purpose the behavior is serving. If you enjoy a glass of wine with dinner, that's one thing, but if you need that glass of wine and don't have any other outlets, I suggest you start searching for some. Consistently seeking an external solution robs you of the satisfaction that comes with filling yourself up with more meaningful ones.

A great way to end a stressful day is to either go to a restorative yoga class or find a quiet space and practice a few poses. You can easily find 20-minute instructional yoga videos for stress relief on YouTube and other video channels.

Other ways to numb

I recently found myself in New Orleans helping my daughter move into a house. Perhaps like you, I have become an expert furniture mover and box packer over the years. My husband moved her once, and I'm on my fourth move. (Her sophomore year dorm room was on the fourth floor of a building with no elevator.) She has moved herself a couple of times, too, which speaks to her sense of independence and empowerment.

As sweat poured off my face, I could almost taste the mold from the bathrooms I'd been scrubbing, and my daughter was telling me for the thousandth time I needed to "be more chill."

Later that evening, she told me that many of her friends' mothers are high when they are in town helping their daughters move. She informed me that one mom drank a lot of wine, another smoked weed, and one of the other women did mushrooms. No wonder they seemed so "chill" as they lugged boxes up four flights of stairs, scrubbed toilets, and hung curtains. I would have been too.

I'm not judging. I get it. Many of these mothers work full-time jobs, have several children, volunteer, and have hectic travel and social schedules.

While I was in my corporate job, I started a habit of drinking wine with my husband most nights while we were preparing dinner. Granted, it was only one glass each evening, but it became a ritual, and I began to find myself looking forward to it and occasionally having a second glass. I justified it by telling myself that there was nothing wrong with what I was doing and that everyone I knew did it too.

The problem is that I had an unsettled feeling about the reason I was having that glass of wine. If I was being honest, I was looking to that wine for comfort. I knew that this behavior did not align with my innermost values.

Plus, I noticed it was interfering with my sleep.

I still have an occasional glass of wine but I have discovered that by giving myself nature breaks during the day, reaching out to friends on a regular basis, practicing 30 minutes of yoga a few times a week, taking time to rest in the evenings, and cuddling with my dogs, I am getting the relief I need.

One of the downsides of using substances to numb – particularly alcohol and marijuana – is the potential to lose inhibitions around food. We are more likely to eat with abandon when we've had a few drinks or smoked pot. For overeaters this leads to extreme guilt after they've sobered up and realize how much and what they ate.

Keep in mind, when I discuss substances, I am not referring to prescription medication you might be taking for a mental health diagnosis. There is a high rate of depression, anxiety, obsessive-compulsive disorder (OCD), attention deficit hyperactivity disorder (ADHD), and other mood disorders among those who overeat. Taking medicine as prescribed is critical to your health.

Purchasing power

Most of us love browsing our favorite online sites to find deals. Sometimes we just like having a stylish new pair of pants or trendy shoes. For others, it can be a compulsion.

When that package from our favorite store arrives on our doorstep, it can even feel exhilarating. In some ways it's similar to the temporary positive sensation you get when consuming the first few bites of a piece of chocolate cake or drinking a Cosmopolitan. I've found that for many clients, shopping can also be a way to achieve a state of numbness, procrastinate, and distract.

And it's so easy. We are just a few clicks away from having what we want appear at our doorstep in a couple of days. It's a quick and immediate sense of pleasure.

Unfortunately, it's also an external feel-good that doesn't last and can lead to a false sense of happiness. It can also result in guilt, shame, and stress if we know deep down that we are buying things for the wrong reasons or spending too much money.

It's so easy to keep going for more stuff. The hard part is to pause long enough to notice what it is you are trying to find in that purchase. What is it that would truly satisfy you from the inside out if it's not that purse you thought you had to have? This is particularly challenging if you have been living in high freeze for years and are completely disconnected with what gives your life meaning and joy.

Parenting to the max

I have found that many parents run themselves ragged trying to make sure their children are exposed to every opportunity available to them. Parents are feeling the pressure to do everything in their power to help their children succeed. It's a vicious cycle that begins with signing them up for a lot of activities that the parents then have to juggle. The result of this lifestyle is an unrelenting frenzied pace that has become the norm for a lot of families.

I refer to this phenomenon as family life in high freeze. The entire family system is taken hostage by busyness, and there is no time to just chill together. Both the parents and children are overwhelmed – maybe even burned out – and everyone is desperately seeking relief from food, drugs, alcohol, technology, or some other self-preserving behavior.

We are living in scary times which the news reminds us of throughout our waking hour. So, it makes sense that parents are doing everything possible to keep their children safe. It's hard not be an anxious parent in today's society. I've seen this translated into parents going to extremes ensuring their children don't have to experience any pain or hardship. Again, this is understandable behavior given the world around us.

Unfortunately, the effort to keep our children from experiencing discomfort in their lives can cause stress for everyone involved.

It's understandable that we want our children to succeed and stay safe, but it's taking a toll on the parents who in their relentless quest to do both are stressed to the max.

Again, I'm not suggesting you stop helping your children or trying to protect them from danger, but instead that you consider the cost vs. benefit of some of the things you are doing for them. For example, if you visit them in college and find yourself doing things they could be doing for themselves and not taking any time for yourself, consider carving out some time for yourself while there. Plan ahead to have a morning to just chill in your hotel room or an afternoon by the pool. It's the same as the oxygen mask on the airplane analogy – you need to take care of yourself if you're going to be any good for them.

Punishing yourself through exercise

Don't take this the wrong way. Exercise is good, especially for stress relief and for your overall health and well-being.

We are bombarded by constant information about exercise. It seems that the messages change almost daily. First it's "you need an hour of aerobic exercise a day for heart health," and then its "you only need 150 minutes a week" or "moderate cardio is OK – wait now it's not enough – you need to have an elevated heart rate for x amount of minutes." It's enough to make your head spin.

If what you are doing is working for you and is sustainable, then no worries.

If you loathe the exercise you're doing, you may not be able to stick with it. Plus being stressed while you're doing it could be counterproductive.

If you go to hot yoga and hate it, ask yourself why you decided to do hot yoga. Did you switch from regular yoga because you heard the hot version burned more calories or because you thought it would build muscle faster? Are you miserable doing hot yoga? Do you see yourself continuing to do hot yoga over the long term?

If you go to a gym but can't stand being on a treadmill under fluorescent lights next to a woman who looks like she works out three hours a day, ask yourself why you are going and what you're getting out of it. If you berate yourself while you're there, that's not good either.

With the right support, some people can find peace with going to the gym. I worked with a client who learned to reframe her negative thoughts about herself at the gym into positive affirmations. She learned to focus on the reasons why she chose to be there and how good she felt when she participated in certain classes.

If your experience at the gym or other form of exercise is more negative than positive, you may want to explore other options for moving your body. Try to think of what you enjoyed as a child before you became body conscious.

Was it biking or swimming, spending time in nature, or dancing? Enlist a friend who wants to ride bikes with you or join you for water aerobics or a Zumba class. Ballroom dancing or creative movement classes can be fun too. Let your inner child out and remember it's okay to look silly.

Achieving to the max

Being an overachiever can be a gift. It means you check items off your to-do list pretty quickly and get a lot accomplished in a day. You likely operate under the assumption that more is better and that you cannot be successful unless you are being productive 24/7, but if you're like many of the women I've counseled, there can be a dark side to this way of life.

A lot of overachievers struggle with finding balance and giving themselves time to rest and restore. They may be operating in high freeze and completely unaware of the toll it's taking on them and others in their life.

If you are an overachiever and you are content, finding time for yourself and things that make you happy, and you are not turning to substances or using self-destructive behaviors to find relief, then there's no reason to consider changing your life.

But if you take some time to assess your life and seek honest input from loved ones or colleagues, you may be surprised at what you discover. They may have been seeing what you were too busy to notice – that you are one stressed out miserable person.

It's no wonder you are overeating or turning to self-preserving behaviors.

CHAPTER 3: Why do smart, successful people do this stuff?

You are likely an intelligent, educated, and highly competent person, although you probably would be the last to acknowledge it. So why would you waste your time numbing yourself when you could be enjoying life?

Why are you standing in your closet every morning berating yourself or taking up space in your head obsessing about the size of your jeans or drinking a bottle of wine every night?

Trying to survive

Generations ago, our ancestors lived in survival mode. Men spent their days in the treacherous wild hunting and gathering to feed their families. Women were responsible for everything else: taking care of the children, preparing food, and tending to the home and relatives and others in the village.

They were stressed, but for different reasons. It was more day-to-day stress. They experienced fear, but often it was in response to a particular event, like being face to face with a tiger. They were busy, but they likely went to bed at sundown. They had no time to pursue pleasure. They had to be skilled at things like basket weaving, cooking, and sewing to provide for their daily needs.

Days started at sunup and ended at sunset. Life revolved around the seasons and the weather. There was little extra time or energy left to ruminate over what might happen tomorrow or what took place years ago. Life was very much in the moment.

Although it seems like we have no time, we actually have a lot more than our ancestors did. We have more hours in the day thanks to electricity. We also have technology to keep our brains stimulated 24/7. So, we have become experts at filling up that extra space with thoughts, worries, activities, and planning.

Our ancestors would probably think we have lost our minds if they could live a day in our shoes. Why would we add more to our days and nights when we could rest? What they would have given for an hour of peace, a short spell to simply do nothing.

We have done such a great job of finding ways to ill up all the hours of the day and night that we have overloaded our circuits, gone against our very nature. The stress is so much that we have become desperate for relief.

Most of the clients I see – intelligent, high-achieving women – do what they do to try to preserve their sanity. The doughnuts in the break room help them cope with the daily onslaught of emails. The ice cream at the end of the day provides a comforting refuge from the chaos. If we had been trained in mindfulness, emotional regulation, self-care, coping tools, and stress management starting in grade school and had parents who modeled these behaviors, we might not have turned to self-destructive ones.

One of my clients was a respected businesswoman in her community. She would function at a high level all day and then hit the bars at night, drink several drinks, overeat high-fat, fried bar food – since she hadn't touched food all day – and get so drunk a friend would have to drive her home. She would start over the next day and do the same. She functioned like this for years until one of her good friends confronted her and insisted she get help.

What's truly amazing is the ability many women have to keep it together at work or for others despite a high level of stress or even trauma. We might practice some level of self-care – like getting regular manicures or massages – but in most cases we need more than just an hour at the spa once a month.

Burnout or putting yourself last

Since most of us live in high freeze, we don't recognize we've gone over the edge until after it's happened. We keep at that daily grind, even tout it as a badge of honor. Like many of you, even though I am sensitive to stress, I can withstand a lot of it. I usually end up hitting the wall multiple times before I decide to make a change. Part of this is because of my tendency to blame myself when things go wrong.

If you're a woman, particularly a mid-career professional, you've probably experienced the symptoms of burnout for years.

Burnout is characterized by the following symptoms:

- Obvious changes in personal habits, such as eating, sleeping, or sex drive
- Cluttered thinking and feeling confused, helpless, overwhelmed, and frustrated
- Negativity, cynicism, and pessimism
- Unable to find pleasure in activities you once enjoyed
- Increased irritability, anger, hostility, or anxiety
- Increased depression
- Increased substance use, including food, alcohol, and drugs
- Difficulty concentrating
- Decreased productivity
- Unmotivated to get out of bed in the morning to face normal daily activities
- Desire to run away from your circumstances
- Longing for things to be different

At one time in my career, my staff consisted of several women in their mid to late 20s and early 30s – in other words millennials. These women had no problems being assertive and asking for what they needed. They were particularly good at taking time off to rest, play, or spend time with loved ones. They also set clear boundaries about how much they were willing to work outside of the office.

I remember feeling resentful as they took vacations to exotic places, and I was stuck at the office. I rarely took time off since it seemed that one of them was always gone, and I thought I had to be there to make sure everything ran smoothly. I had convinced myself I didn't have a choice.

While it was true that someone needed to be available when they were gone, I realize I could have probably taken more vacation time too. I had allowed myself to become a martyr/victim and was also setting a standard for the rest of my staff that was not healthy. When I finally started taking more time off, I was less stressed, and my staff was relieved to know I was human.

What I realized later was that this group of women taught me invaluable lessons about self-care and work-life balance.

I'm not saying all millennials have the option that these women did – in fact many of you are struggling financially and burdened with debt, but I try to remember what I learned from this particular group of women – that self-care and work-life balance is important.

I had a colleague recently tell me that after taking only a week off it took her three weeks to catch up with all the emails and projects she missed. For many, it feels as if it's not worth going on vacation, since the workload you face upon returning is so overwhelming. Some feel pressure to keep up with work while away. I used to be guilty of that until I realized I just needed to set clear boundaries and take advantage of voicemail and email notifications saying I was out of the office.

In some work situations, it seems impossible to find work-life balance. I still think it's important to ask yourself: Am I taking on more than I need to? Are there any tasks I could delegate? Is there any part of me that is playing the martyr or victim? Do I have any unresolved feelings about letting go of some of the responsibilities? What about taking time off? How do I feel about slowing down? Ultimately, another question to ask yourself is if another job might be healthier for you.

We allow our pets to rest and our children to nap, but we ignore our own needs for time to restore.

Several recent studies have shown the importance of downtime for increased creativity, connection, inner peace, inspiration, and even productivity. I've found that taking this last year to work from home, setting aside time to take mindful walks in my yard, watch and listen to the birds, or just play with my dogs is what allowed me to write this book. The empty space is what got my creative juices going.

As I was writing this book, I kept thinking I should be doing more. This wasn't enough. It wasn't going to happen fast enough. It wasn't going to lead to the financial success that I need to pay our bills and save for retirement. My worry about money kept creeping in and casting a dark cloud over my desire to write. Instead of allowing myself to be in the moment and let the organic process flow, I found myself going back to the numbers in my bank account. It was uncomfortable, even painful at times, but I'm glad I stuck with it. I've fulfilled a dream. And that feels good.

The elusive self-esteem

In my moments of doubt and insecurity when I am convinced I cannot be successful again, my business coach Gail looks at me sternly and says, "What makes you think you can't, Beth?"

We are all born with a sense of self-esteem. It's what happens next that either boosts it or eats away at it.

In a perfect world, our every need is attended to and our every emotion is validated. We are fed when we are hungry, changed when our diapers are dirty, held and comforted when we are sad, and told that all of our emotions are OK to have, but this certainly isn't always the case, so we figure out how to adapt. If we have fewer needs, then we won't be disappointed if they aren't met. If we invalidate our own needs, then we can avoid thinking that our caregivers are doing a lousy job. When we are young and dependent, we have to think our caregivers are good, because we can't survive without them. Instead of blaming our parents, we believe there is something wrong with us. So, our self-esteem decreases as an adaptation to our environment.

We become adults who think we aren't worthy, and that's how we relate in the world, and our self-concept seems to fluctuate depending on the environment. We might feel OK in certain situations or around certain people – supportive friends who validate our emotions, for instance, or in nature or with a trusted dog – but then down in the dirt when we're with certain family members who bring up those little girl thoughts of not being good enough.

You can't change your family of origin or anyone else, but you can learn tools to improve your self-esteem. I like to refer to it as developing your own healthy inner parent. You can learn how to give yourself what your parents were not able to offer. If you don't have supportive people in your life, a good place to turn is to a therapist, life coach or mentor. I also recommend support groups for the healing power of being surrounded by others who are in the same boat as you.

Reflect:

What are some people, situations, or environments that may have contributed to your low self-esteem?

Observe:

What might you need in your life to improve your self-esteem? Notice what emotions and body sensations come up when you think about this need.

Reach:

Talk to a safe support person about how you might begin to ill this need. Ask them to hold you accountable for doing what you say you are going to do – this may mean making an appointment with a therapist or life coach or joining a support group.

Trying something different

By now, you may already have had an "aha" moment as to why you keep trying to find relief in sweet, starchy, or fatty foods. You could also probably list your symptoms, but here goes a cheat sheet.

Signs that you have a problem with overeating may include:

- Years of weight fluctuations
- Digestive issues, acid reflux
- Spending a lot of time and money on health, food, body, and/or appearance
- Saying to yourself, "I shouldn't be eating because I'm fat"
- Constantly searching for the latest health or diet fad, such as plant-based dieting
- Eating small amounts of "good" food in public, secretive eating of "bad" foods
- Guilt after eating
- Constantly comparing yourself to others and coming up short

- Isolating from friends, family, or colleagues
- Work problems, difficulty focusing
- Feeling irritable, depressed, or anxious
- Low self-esteem
- Feeling hopeless or stuck
- Intimacy problems
- Not taking time for yourself or for activities you enjoy
- Feeling compelled to drink alcohol or use marijuana or other nonprescription drugs almost daily
- Can't get off the sofa to exercise
- Can't take a day off from exercising, you feel compelled to exercise to burn calories
- Bouncing back and forth between eating "healthy" and exercising and eating "unhealthy" and not exercising
- Trouble sleeping
- Shame

I hear you saying, "But I have so many of these – it's hopeless" or "I have so much going on in my life, I don't have time to deal with all this" or "It's too late – I'm too old to change." I've also heard many clients say, "I feel so stupid. I should have dealt with this years ago."

Try to remind yourself that you really have been doing all you could to stay afloat. If you're reading this, you are likely sick and tired of living this way which means you're ready to change.

I get that having to do one more thing to try to end your overeating may feel overwhelming, but if you have even a seed of willingness to try something different, then you will succeed. You may be scared and untrusting, but there's something in you that is encouraging you to take the leap.

Your time is now.

SECTION 2: Why can't I stop?

CHAPTER 4: Eating behaviors are complicated

Overeating stems from a complex interplay of the brain, hormones, and the environment.

Restrictive dieting alone can turn a normal eater into an overeater in a matter of weeks. I often hear from clients or workshop participants that they are addicted to food, particularly white flour and sugar, and that the only times they have been able to temporarily stop overeating is when they've eliminated these foods from their diet.

The problem with the abstinence approach is that it's not sustainable for most people. In fact, it's near impossible. I'm not saying it's easy to live a life that incorporates these types of food without overdoing it, but if you follow my recommendations, you will eventually be able to eat these foods in moderation. I like to refer to it as building the moderation mindset muscle.

Does this sound like you?

- You are emotionally sensitive, though you tend to internalize your emotions rather than expressing them.

- You find yourself more sensitive to stress than friends and colleagues.

- You tend to be the responsible one, a caretaker of the world.

- You are a people pleaser who puts everyone else's needs before yours.

- You suffer from low self-esteem.
- You have difficulty being assertive and setting boundaries with friends, colleagues, and family.
- You have a harsh inner critic, constantly beating yourself up or yelling at yourself.

The overeating brain

If you are prone to overeating, then you likely have lower-than-normal dopamine D2 receptors in the part of your brain called the striatum. It also means you have decreased inhibitions, or less self-control, around food.[14]

Dopamine is a naturally occurring chemical in the body that acts as a neurotransmitter and neurohormone. While it is commonly associated with reward and pleasure, it also has a role regulating movement, memory, hormones, and even pregnancy. Some studies have linked binge eating disorder to a hyperresponsiveness to rewards such as food, which means eating is more rewarding and produces more pleasure in these individuals.[15] Research has shown that binge eating also is associated with release of dopamine in certain parts of the brain.[16]

The "big three" hormones

Ghrelin: An easy way to think of ghrelin is as the "hungry" hormone. Ghrelin is a hormone that regulates our appetite and also plays a role in body weight.

Ghrelin helps our bodies defend against stress. When we are stressed, our ghrelin levels increase, which results in a stronger drive for food. It also means the food we eat tastes better. When our ghrelin level is high, then our dopamine also goes up, which means food becomes more rewarding – and this can result in compulsive eating. The more ghrelin, the more hunger, and since dieting is stressful, it can cause increases in ghrelin.

Leptin: If ghrelin is hungry, then think of leptin as the "full" hormone. Leptin, made by fat cells, also helps regulate appetite by letting us know when we are full. When you lose weight, the weight loss itself results in decreased leptin, which means it takes more food to feel full.

Under normal circumstances, your fat cells release leptin into the bloodstream, which in turn tells your body there is enough energy stored and signals your body to eat less. When you diet and lose fat, your leptin decreases, which leads to increased appetite as the body attempts to bump up its energy stores.

So, weight loss actually leads to increased hunger. This is one of the many reasons it is hard to lose pounds and keep them off. It is not a lost cause; it just means that restrictive dieting is not the answer.

Cortisol: We have started to hear more about this hormone in recent years. Cortisol is what we refer to as the stress hormone. It's basically our body's way of notifying us when we're under stress, and it works with certain parts of the brain to regulate our moods, motivation, and fear.

Cortisol is made by the adrenal glands and is best known as the "fight, flight, or freeze" hormone. What a lot of people don't realize is that chronic, unrelenting high levels of stress can also lead to high blood sugar, weight gain, problems with sleep, digestive issues, headaches, cardiovascular problems, and increased anxiety and depression.

Notice weight gain is on that list. So once again, if dieting results in stress, which increases cortisol, then it's going to be hard to lose weight without gaining it back, and it makes sense that negative body image would also add to stress levels and thus higher cortisol, as one study suggests.[17] Additional research has demonstrated that painful exercise increases stress, while enjoyable exercise decreases cortisol.[18][19][20][21]

Polycystic ovary syndrome (PCOS)

According to the U.S. Department of Health and Human Services' Office on Women's Health, polycystic ovary syndrome affects 1 in 10 women of childbearing age. PCOS is a condition caused by an imbalance in the hormones in your brain and ovaries, and it can start at any age after puberty. PCOS often isn't detected until a woman tries to get pregnant and discovers she has fertility issues. Symptoms include cravings for high-fat, sugar-laden food, irregular menses, unexplained weight gain in the abdomen, excess facial hair, thinning hair on the head, and darkening skin or skin tags.[22]

Unfortunately, many women with PCOS not only suffer needlessly but end up being bullied and blamed for their sugar cravings and weight gain. In my experience, these same girls and women begin to believe they are responsible for not being able to control their eating or weight, which leads to shame and thoughts that something is wrong with them. This in turn results in behaviors like hiding the foods they crave, eating them in secret, and eventually bingeing and even purging.

One of the first questions I ask my female clients is about their menstrual history and food cravings. Often, I'll hear that they had irregular menses from the start and that they craved sweets, carbs, and high-fat foods as children. I ask if they've struggled with weight in their midsection or if they've ever had unwanted hair on their face or torso. If they respond with a resounding "yes," then I recommend they get tested for PCOS by their internist or OB-GYN.

Untreated PCOS can result in years of struggling with food cravings and a lot of misplaced shame and blame. I had one client who craved sugar and carbs as a child. Her mother constantly tried to limit her intake of sweets, but the girl ended up hiding them in her room and bingeing on them.

Her mother did what most concerned mothers would and took her to the family doctor. Since the girl had started gaining weight, the doctor did what most doctors would have at the time and recommended a diet.

Unfortunately, this approach set my client up for years of secretive eating that morphed into bingeing and eventual excessive weight gain, which led to severe negative body image and low self-esteem.

After meeting with her once and reviewing her childhood history, I suggested she get evaluated for PCOS which it turned out she had. Discovering that there was a medical explanation for her food cravings and struggles with weight lifted some of the shame and sense of powerlessness she felt since childhood. She was able to get on medicine and, with therapy, stop the vicious cycle of bingeing and body shaming.

I often ask my clients how their overeating has served them and what else they might have turned to if it hadn't been food.

For many, the eating spared them from developing even more self-destructive behaviors, such as the overuse of drugs or alcohol. This is why I started referring to overeating as a type of self-preservation.

Overeating behaviors

When I present the following information, I usually hear "But I do all of these" or "I don't exactly it into any of these categories." I'm used to working with perfectionists and overachievers, so I'll let you in on a secret: It's OK. Labeling your disordered eating behavior is not nearly as important as understanding how and why it started, why you continue to turn to it, and learning how to stop doing it.

Binge eating: Most people think of binge eating as someone sitting in front of a television gorging on ice cream, cookies, and chips until they are so stuffed, they can't move. This is a fairly apt description, although not everyone who binges does so with sweets or carbs. I've actually had clients who binge on carrots and veggies. The key is that the person eats a large quantity of food, experiences a loss of control, and might feel guilt or distress after eating. Often, when someone refers to themselves as a binge eater, they aren't. Since there is a lot of misinformation out there about what a person should consume in a day – calories, for instance, or types or amounts of food – it is easy to get confused and think you are binge eating. I've even worked with clients who insist that eating a piece of cake is a binge. What differentiates binge eating from a full-blown binge eating disorder is that for the clinical diagnosis the person binges at least once a week and has done so for three consecutive months.

Compulsive eating: Compulsive eaters typically ingest small amounts of food throughout the day or night. Some refer to it as "grazing." They tend to constantly be thinking of food – when or what they will eat next is always on their mind. If there is no actual reward from compulsive eating, why would an intelligent, capable person keep doing it? Consistently turning to food represents an attempt to manage negative emotions, such as stress, anger, frustration, irritability, dread, sadness, hopelessness, grief, or fatigue. If you think about it, it's an understandable distraction.

I remember my senior year in college when I was living by myself in an apartment in downtown Palo Alto, California. I was loaded up with 20 credit hours each semester to make up for my year in Italy, where I ended up foregoing school the entire spring semester. Since I chose to study alone in my apartment, I would munch on trail mix and chips as I poured over my books. I would end up with practically debilitating stomachaches each time, but that didn't stop me from continuing the behavior.

I had a client who had an extremely stressful job working for an overpowering boss in a chaotic office setting. She was bombarded with phone calls all day, and when she wasn't on the phone her boss was standing in her office demanding that she take on another project. She was in such a hurry to get to work early to please her boss that she would skip breakfast, but she always made sure to have a drawerful of snacks in her desk. Grazing on those sweet, salty, crunchy foods helped her get through the day.

The problem with this behavior is that the food only provides short-term relief and can cause a lot of physical discomfort and long-term weight gain. It can also be expensive. Many of my clients who eat compulsively will stock up on items they can stash away at the office or in a secret location in their house, so they always have easy access to their go-to foods.

Stress-induced eating: Stress eating is exactly what it sounds like. It makes sense, especially now that you know there are both biological – remember that our hunger hormone, ghrelin, increases in response to stress – and psychological reasons for craving that chocolate after a fight with your partner or a long day at the office. High levels of stress alter our hormones, setting us up to crave certain foods, mainly those that are sugary, salty, and fatty. Stress actually makes these foods taste even better.[23]

Night eating: Many binge/emotional eaters tend to skimp on their portions during the day, either because they don't take the time to eat meals or when they do eat with others, they have excessive anxiety about being seen eating anything other than a salad. These types of eaters tend to go straight to a drive-through, convenience store, or grocery store and binge on their way home or sit in front of the TV and eat continuously until bedtime.

Night eating syndrome, on the other hand, is a diagnosable illness and includes restricting intake for most of the day and then consuming most of your food in the evening or at night. Those with night eating syndrome – it's diagnosed if the behavior has occurred for at least three months – often have mood and sleep disorders.

Many people with this disorder feel a tremendous amount of shame because they think it is their fault and that there is something wrong with them. They beat themselves up for the weight gain that inevitably comes with not eating during the day and eating a lot at night. It is hard to talk about, so they typically don't tell their healthcare providers – so when their weight continues to creep up on the scale, so does their shame and sense of helplessness. If you think you may have this condition, consult your doctor and ask to be referred to an eating disorder specialist.

The "ultraclean eater"

I prefer to eat whole foods that don't have a lot of chemicals in them. Growing up, we had butter in the fridge instead of margarine and cooked food from scratch. We also ate lots of fresh fruits and vegetables. The down side was that we rarely had treats or snacks available.

As soon as my daughter could sit up, I put her on the counter and had her help me add flour and butter to the cookie recipes. One of my greatest joys is that she not only knows how to cook for herself but actually derives pleasure in the process.

I am certainly a proponent of eating organic when possible, supporting local farmers and providing my body with the nutrients it needs to feel good and have energy. I see problems arise when my clients take healthy eating to the extreme. Their decision to eliminate all "unhealthy" foods may align with their value of saving the planet or preventing disease, but it could also increase their stress level since they have to spend a lot of time, energy, and money planning their meals. There's also the problem of trying to do it perfectly with the intention of never eating foods that aren't in their regimen. Lastly, there's the risk of overeating foods that aren't considered "clean" and/or feeling compelled to find ways to purify after consuming these foods.

What I often see with clean eaters is a sense of isolation since they tend to avoid activities they used to enjoy like eating out in certain restaurants, having dinner at a friend's house, or traveling. Their dietary restrictions tend to take up a lot of time and energy and can also be stressful on others in their life.

Recently, a colleague invited me to attend a seminar on plant-based eating. The presenter was a local physician.

The room was filled with therapists, dietitians, and others interested in the topic. The doctor had recently been certified in integrative medicine, and she was excited to share information from her program. She showed slide after slide full of evidence that eating a plant-based diet could reverse certain diseases and prevent others. The diet she proposed was based on plant-based foods as your entire source of nutrients. No meat. No dairy. No gluten and no fat other than a few tablespoons of olive oil a week.

I am not here to dispute the validity of the research on plant-based eating for health purposes or for the well-being of the planet. I just know that "in the wrong brain" this could be taken to an unhealthy extreme. I've seen too many start the journey and end up feeling isolated, unhappy, stressed, and of course eventually bingeing on the foods they tried to eliminate. I've also seen people adopt strict dietary approaches who end up slipping into other unhealthy behaviors in an attempt to find pleasure in their lives.

Orthorexia

The term orthorexia nervosa is not an official diagnosis in the Diagnostic and Statistical Manual of Mental Disorders, but it is a potentially serious condition that warrants discussion.

From the Greek, the term literally means "correct diet," which sounds healthy and benign.

But those living with orthorexia exhibit an unhealthy obsession with the quality of foods they consume. In the case of these individuals, quantity is generally not the issue. Many who are obsessed with this hyper version of clean eating also display disordered eating behaviors. I have seen a lot of people with anorexia who have orthorexia, but I am also seeing more people with overeating behaviors who have become obsessed with maintaining pure bodies.

The behavior may start off with a desire to eat healthier, but over time the person adopts a highly restrictive lifestyle that excludes most foods other than certain vegetables. Certain foods and nutrients are even idealized as having magical healing qualities – think kale and chlorella – and these people begin to believe that eating these foods and eliminating others is a badge of honor. People with orthorexia become distressed at even the thought of eating foods that are not in their repertoire, and they may even show disgust when eating around others who are consuming these foods.

Orthorexia is often paired with obsessive exercise, which means the person has essentially become a machine whose entire life revolves around what they eat and how much they exercise. The seeking out, preparing, and consuming of these foods is almost ritualistic. Orthorexia nervosa usually goes unnoticed because it does not seem unusual today to be focused on healthy eating and exercise. What's particularly disturbing is that not only do these extreme behaviors go unchecked – even by healthcare professionals – but the person may be malnourished and at risk of a serious medical complication, such as anemia, low blood pressure, an electrolyte abnormality, or osteoporosis.

Some signs that you or a loved one may have orthorexia:

- A sense of accomplishment and even elation from clean, healthy, pure eating.

- Excessive time spent thinking about, planning for, and consuming food.

- Guilt when consuming foods that are not considered healthy and pure.

- Anxiety when meals are not planned in advance.

- Judging or having critical thoughts about others who choose not to eat pure, healthy foods.

- Avoiding eating out or traveling to places where you can't get the foods you think you need. Having to prepare your own meals at home. No longer going out to eat with friends or loved ones or enjoying holiday meals.

- Insisting on bringing food to others' homes when you're invited over for a meal.

- Symptoms of depression, anxiety, irritability, mood swings, shame, or guilt.

- Refusing to eat in restaurants or with others due to food restrictions and a need to be in control of food preparation.

- Increased isolation and disconnectedness.

Reflect:

Write a list of all the things you did and enjoyed before the obsession with clean eating took over your life – activities, places you went, people you hung out with, and foods.

Observe:

What do you miss about these things? How do you think your life might be improved by returning to some of these former activities? Ask yourself if this new lifestyle is aligned with your authentic values. Does clean eating bring you closer to what you value or farther from the things that give your life meaning?

Reach:

If you conclude that some of your eating behaviors are interfering with your life or have become unhealthy, I recommend you share your concerns with a friend or loved one and seek professional help.

But I'm addicted to certain foods

This is a hot topic that is quite controversial. While there is evidence to show that certain foods are addictive – and the food industry has spent millions of dollars developing hyperpalatable foods to make sure we salivate at the mere thought of them[24] – the problem is that it's almost impossible to live according to the abstinence model. It is a setup for failure.

I've worked with countless people who insist they can't eat sugar or bread, for example. I had a client who recently informed me that if she eats one piece of bread, she will finish the loaf.

I get it. I used to have the same problem with foods like pizza, popcorn, cookies, chips, and ice cream. It took me years to be able to eat any of these foods without bingeing on them. I've yet to work with an overeater who was able to successfully abstain from these so-called "addictive" foods for the long term unless they replaced them with other substances or self-destructive behaviors.

You may not be sold on the idea that you will be able to eat the foods you crave in moderation. I'm not asking for a vote of confidence, just that you be willing to consider that it's possible. All you have to do is keep reading and put one foot in front of the other. The main ingredients for success are persistence and practice.

Note: If you after reading this chapter, you think you might have a full-blown eating disorder; please seek professional help with an eating disorder specialist. Your doctor should be able to refer you to one in your community. You can find free eating disorder screenings and referral sources online. A good place to start is the National Eating Disorders Association or NEDA.

CHAPTER 5: Disordered eating does not discriminate

Men and disordered eating

I began to see a pattern with the men I treated over the years. Many of the men who ended up struggling with their weight and developing disordered eating patterns had either been born into larger bodies, started puberty early or been bullied for their size. Some of the men had been high school athletes who gained a lot of weight during their freshman year in college and began the cycle of restricting and overeating after that.

I had an adult male client who had experienced abandonment as a child. He turned to sweets for comfort and struggled with his weight and being bullied at school. He was determined to lose weight in high school and started dieting.

He ended up in my office because he was tired of living this way and ready to change. Therapy helped him understand that the bingeing had been his way of coping with his childhood abandonment and the bullying. After only a few months of following the protocol outlined in the coming chapters, he was able to stop bingeing and live a life free of obsession about food, weight, and his body.

Boys and men are feeling the pressure to have perfect bodies too. I've worked with young men whose eating and body issues began innocently with trying to get it and bulk up. In their attempt to have perfectly sculpted physiques, these males may become obsessed with clean eating, and for those prone to overeating, the vicious cycle of restricting and dieting begins.

Although about 3 million American men suffer from full-blown binge eating disorder, the majority of them do not seek help. Many fear being stigmatized, since our culture projects the idea that anything to do with food, weight, and mental health is a female issue. Some also fear being labeled homosexual, since they believe a societal misconception that only gay men have issues with food and body image. In fact, studies have shown that while a larger number of gay men do seek treatment for eating disorders, the majority of men with eating disorders are not gay.

LGBTQ+ and disordered eating

LGBTQ+ people face a unique set of challenges that may put them at greater risk of developing disordered eating and body image issues. Elevated rates of binge eating and purging by vomiting or laxative abuse has been found for people who identified as gay, lesbian, bisexual or "mostly heterosexual" in comparison to heterosexuals.

Some factors that place people at a higher risk for disordered eating and full-blown eating disorders occur at higher rates in the LGBTQ+ community. Exposure to oppression, discrimination, homophobia, and transphobia often lead to high rates of depression, anxiety, and even trauma, which contribute to the risk of developing severe issues with eating and body image.

Other contributing factors to disordered eating for LGBTQ+ people:

- Experiences of being bullied
- Experiences of violence due to their sexual orientation or gender identity
- Lack of support from family or the community where they were raised
- Feeling different and left out

- Pressure to achieve the body ideals of the LGBTQ+ community
- Long-term effects of stress and discrimination
- Unsafe home environment
- Fear of rejection by friends, family, and coworkers
- Internalized negative messages

Transgender people, specifically, have their own set of complicating factors. Since transgender people experience gender dysphoria – discomfort with their biological sex – the result for many is negative body image and extreme uneasiness with their bodies. This is a strong foundation for developing disordered eating or full-blown eating disorders.

Together, these factors suggest the risk of eating disorders could be higher for LGBTQ+ people. It is well documented that the rates of depression, anxiety, trauma, and substance abuse are higher among LGBTQ+ individuals as a result of these stressors. Studies of LBGTQ+ people with disordered eating are limited, but some have shown that transgender people seem to have the highest rates of disordered eating when compared to other LGBTQ+ people and people who are cis-gendered heterosexual, someone whose gender identity matches their biological sex.[25][26][27] Research in 2009 found that during adolescence, girls who identify as lesbian, bisexual, or "mostly heterosexual" and boys who identify as gay, bisexual, or "mostly heterosexual" have higher rates of binge eating and purging than their heterosexual peers.[28]

If you identify as a member of the LGBTQ+ community and are struggling with disordered eating, you may have some qualms about seeking help. Be sure to ask any professional what their experience is working with LGBTQ+ clients; if they haven't had any experience, you sense any hesitation in their voice, or any hint of discrimination, then I suggest you look for someone else.

Race and ethnicity issues

People from all racial and ethnic backgrounds struggle with food and body image issues, disordered eating, and full-blown eating disorders.

Every ethnicity and race seem to have their own messages about food and weight. Some cultures historically encourage eating a lot of food (Italian) and seem to celebrate larger bodies and curves (African American and Latinx), while other cultures are hyper-focused on showing restraint and keeping your waistline in check (Asian), but the lines are becoming blurred. The diet industry, clothing industry, and media are targeting everyone, everywhere, and as we know, simply starting a diet can set off the chemical reaction for developing disordered eating or full-blown eating disorders.

Some healthcare providers overlook the differences inherent in diverse races and ethnicities as they relate to disordered eating, since many of these providers are still under the impression it's a "white girl's disease." These same providers are likely to recommend a diet to a larger-sized African American woman who has the exact body she is meant to have and is perfectly healthy based on her BMI.

CHAPTER 6: Diet frenzy

The most purchased type of nonfiction book in America is the diet book.

By now, most of you recognize the diets you have tried have not worked. In fact, all the money you've spent and misery you've put yourself through has likely resulted in more weight gain and feelings of powerlessness or even desperation. The worst part is that instead of pointing the finger at the diet program or the doctor who recommended it to you, you end up blaming yourself for not being able to stick to it.

You may have asked yourself at some point why you keep dieting even though it hasn't helped you keep the weight off for the long term. Some of it has to do with the way the diet industry knows how to get inside your head. They understand that you're unhappy with your weight and that you want to believe there is one last diet that will make you thin forever. They prey on your sense of magical thinking. We are human. We want to believe in fairy tale endings.

Another reason people keep trying new diets is that there's constant talk about the obesity epidemic. It's hard not to feel a sense of urgency.

There are almost daily reports in the media-citing studies linking obesity to serious medical consequences.

While I am not here to dispute that obesity can lead to health problems for some people or that weight loss is wrong, the way the medical community and the media are addressing the problem is causing a lot of stress. It's also led to increased weight phobia and stigma toward those living in bodies that don't meet society's ideal shape or weight.

The standard method for measuring obesity is BMI which does not take into account age, body type, muscle mass vs. body fat, developmental stage, or ethnicity. In recent years disputes about BMI as a measure of health have come under scrutiny. Some argue that there are more accurate measures of health including skinfold thickness, waist to hip circumference, densitometry (underwater weighing), and dual energy X-Ray (Dexa) to name a few.[29]

One thing is certain – the diet industry is thriving in our obesity-focused environment. Now there are even programs aimed specifically at children. If diets worked, then our obesity problem would be solved, and we would be healthier as a population – in mind, body, and spirit. It seems that our society as a whole is caught up in an unrelenting cycle that is only causing more stress and leading to poorer outcomes for everyone but the 60-million-dollar diet industry.

The most startling statistic about dieting is that 95 percent of those who diet actually regain the weight they initially lost; many gain additional weight,[30][31] and up to 2.8 percent of all Americans will develop clinical eating disorders.[32]

Research also found that 35 percent of "normal dieters" eventually turn to nonstop dieting. Of those, up to 25 percent develop disordered eating or full-blown eating disorders.[33] Among girls age 6 to 12, it's estimated that between 40 percent and 50 percent are concerned about their weight and shape, which contributes to potential restrictive eating during such a crucial developmental stage.

In a large study of 14- and 15-year-olds, dieting was the most important predictor of developing an eating disorder. Those who dieted moderately were five times more likely to develop an eating disorder, and those who practiced extreme restriction were eighteen times more likely to develop an eating disorder than those who did not diet.[34]

Here's the down and dirty on dieting: Most people have a limit to the amount of self-control they can exert. It's just mentally exhausting to keep doing what you hate, and unless you live alone on an island, you are constantly bombarded with foods you love.

It's not natural to deprive yourself of what you want for the long term. If you go out with friends for pizza and only allow yourself to eat a salad, you are likely to have pizza on your mind the entire time – and it will only be a matter of time before you end up eating an entire pizza alone in your room. That's why I recommend working toward a moderation mindset with food.

Notice I say "working toward," since this is a long-term process.

The landmark 1950 Minnesota Semi-Starvation Study by Ancel Keys provides invaluable information on the effects of a restricted diet. Thirty-six people agreed to participate in a 6-month restrictive food diet and soon began to exhibit a multitude of behavioral, emotional, and physical changes. Food preoccupation, unusual eating habits, periods of binge eating, extreme emotional distress that included significant depression, wildly fluctuating moods, and irritability were all observed, along with poor concentration, comprehension, and judgment. Participants also showed sleep disruption, gastrointestinal disturbance, and weakness, among other physical ramifications. During the refeeding process, the most common symptom of those in this semi-starved state was binge eating. This study shows the importance of maintaining a consistent source of fuel for your system, including adequate calories, to fend off starvation effects.[35]

A vicious cycle begins with calorie restriction, particularly for those at higher risk for disordered eating, with various impairments aggravating the other. Ongoing research continues to support the findings of the Keys study; it's now widely accepted that impaired brain function can alter mood and affect judgment, behavior, personality, cognition, response flexibility, and autonomic nervous system control. Fluctuating levels of glucose, the brain's primary food, may help explain some of the shifting personality and emotional and other aspects in a dieter's behaviors. Since neurons cannot store glucose, they require a continual supply to the brain; when glucose levels are low, the brain starts to suffer and can show typical hypoglycemic symptoms of shakiness, irritability, hunger, weakness, increased pulse rate, and anxiety.[36]

Most people, when they have low blood sugar, will attempt to address their need by seeking the necessary nutrients. This drive to find food, which generally provides a pleasurable and calming effect, comes from the hypothalamus.[37][38]

Dieting = Stress

The real problem with dieting is that it increases stress levels. All that weighing and measuring and obsessing about everything that goes into your mouth not only wears you out, but it wreaks havoc on hormones like cortisol (the stress hormone), ghrelin (the hunger hormone), and leptin (the hormone that tells you when you're full).

One study on the impact of elevated cortisol demonstrated that increased stress reinforces the value of palatable food – being stressed out actually makes food you already find pleasurable even more enjoyable.[39] Other research has shown that consuming high-fat, sugar-laden foods temporarily reduces your stress level, that such foods increase serotonin and promote a calming effect.[40][41]

In one study, after putting people through emotional and physical stress, those with elevated cortisol levels chose foods with the most fat and carbs.[42]

In the Stress in America survey, commissioned annually by the American Psychological Association, many adults report unhealthy eating behaviors as a result of stress and say these behaviors can lead to undesirable consequences, such as feeling sluggish or lazy or feeling bad about their bodies.

In the most recent study, 38 percent of adults said they had overeaten or eaten unhealthy foods in the past month because of stress. Half of these adults (49 percent) reported engaging in these behaviors at least once a week, and one-third of them said they did so because it helped distract them from the stress.

Twenty-seven percent of adults said they eat to manage stress, and 34 percent of those who reported overeating or eating unhealthy foods because of stress called the behavior a habit.

Thirty percent of adults reported skipping a meal due to stress in the past month, and 41 percent who did so said they did it at least once a week.

The stress of cyclical dieting, weight fluctuations, and self-criticism add fuel to an already raging ire. Stress alters your hormones and intensifies your urge to eat – it literally changes the chemistry of your body. If you are constantly shoulding yourself, your stress only amplifies: "I should eat a salad without dressing for lunch" or "I should cut out all carbs."

Common causes of stress include:

- Adverse childhood experiences (ACEs), such as family conflict, abuse, neglect, abandonment, or invaliding parents

- Trauma
- Sickness or death in the family
- Divorce
- Financial or food insecurity
- Exposure to the news
- Caring for a loved one with addiction, an eating disorder, or mental illness
- Social media or always being "plugged in"
- Lack of sleep
- Dieting and exercise you hate

High levels of stress in general can lead to:

- Drug and alcohol use
- Disordered eating or full-blown eating disorders
- Depression and/or anxiety
- Changes in brain chemistry/hormones
- Our ability to self-regulate or calm ourselves

If you are a stress-sensitive person, you are going to react more intensely to things that others take in stride.

Stress-sensitive individuals actually have a larger amygdala – the part of the brain responsible for fear, anger, vigilance, and, of course, stress – and a smaller hippocampus and prefrontal cortex, the areas of the brain that help manage stress. Chronic stress causes the neurons in the amygdala to grow and strengthen and the neurons in the hippocampus to atrophy and die. A larger amygdala and smaller hippocampus make it more difficult to manage stress.

Seemingly benign or even positive situations can lead to severe distress and extreme behavioral reactions for those who are stress sensitive – things like moving to a new home or city, starting a new job, going on vacation, or meeting new people.

While most people have the ability to tolerate these types of life events, those who are stress sensitive have a much lower threshold. Since we don't have our brains scanned at birth to determine if we are one of those individuals, the chances are pretty good that we aren't aware why we have such extreme reactions – and neither are our friends, loved ones, or coworkers.

Even worse, it's likely you've been given grief or even criticized for how you behave. Many of my clients grew up hearing statements like "that's ridiculous," "you're overreacting," or "you're too sensitive." Over time you begin to believe that you are the problem and invalidate your own inner experience. Instead of opening up to others about how you feel, you keep it all to yourself. Not only that, you criticize yourself, tell yourself you're crazy, and build a stockpile of shame. In order to cope, you turn to numbing behaviors.

You may be stress sensitive if:

- You react strongly to loud noise.
- You have an aversion to scratchy materials.
- You are sensitive to change or have trouble with surprises.
- You are sensitive to others' reactions or feedback.
- Little things get under your skin.

A woman I counseled wanted to know if it was normal that she ate candy all day at work. She had a high-powered job with a large national company, and although she had been there 10 years and was a manager, she rarely took time out during the day to take a break. She would skip breakfast and occasionally eat lunch at her desk – if she even ate lunch. Ironically, she worked in a place where she could get free delicious food any time she wanted.

After learning about the correlation between stress and urges to overeat, she had her "aha" moment. The candy was helping her manage her stress and function. It was like reaching for a drink or a pill to calm her nerves. She worried that without the regular ingestion of candy, she would fall apart at work and not be as productive.

Instead of suggesting that she stop eating candy, we looked at ways she could reduce her stress level at work. She came up with creating a grounding space in her office that contained essential oils and something soft to the touch. She also liked the idea of sipping on a cup of hot tea and taking breaks to walk outside. When she started taking better care of herself, she found she didn't need the candy.

But more is better when it comes to exercise, right?

There really can be too much of a good thing.

In our exercise centric world, there are those who are taking it to the extreme. You know who you are. What likely started out as an innocent way to get in shape, lose weight, or de-stress has completely taken over your life.

Signs you may be taking your exercise program too far:

- The exercise is a daily activity, and taking a day or more off from the gym causes extreme anxiety and/or guilt.
- You exercise even if you are injured or sick. You brave icy roads or other inclement weather or put yourself in dangerous situations like working out late at night or in unsafe neighborhoods alone.

- You consistently disregard work, social, or family activities to exercise. For example, you can't take one night off running to watch a movie with your family.

- You feel compelled to do a certain type of exercise or workout, and if that is not available, you become anxious or irritable.

- Your primary motivation to exercise is to burn calories, lose weight, or reduce your percentage of body fat, and when you don't exercise the amount you think you should, you restrict your caloric intake to compensate.

- You exercise to avoid spending time with others.

- Your self-worth and sense of overall well-being is dependent on how much you exercise.

- You use exercise as a way to avoid unwanted emotions instead of coping with them.

- You find no pleasure in the exercise, and it actually feels abusive or like a form of punishment. You may be in physical or even emotional pain – scared or stressed if a trainer is standing over you screaming to push harder.

I coined the term "steporexia" to describe the step-counting phenomenon that has taken place in recent years. Pedometers have been handed out at work and school, and everyone seems obsessed with reaching 10,000 steps per day, but it turns out that 10,000 was a random number chosen as a marketing strategy.

According to I-Min Lee, the lead author of a new study in the Journal of the American Medical Association, a Japanese company selling pedometers in 1965 gave it a name that, in Japanese, means "the 10,000 step meter." The Japanese researchers chose this name because the character for "10,000" resembles a man walking. According to Lee, the relationship between that number and actual health has never been proven. So, from that randomness, we have all become fixated on 10,000 steps a day. I've had clients of all ages who have been so focused on the number that they stay up late at night just to reach their daily goal.[43]

If you are an overachiever, you might find yourself doing more than you need. If 10,000 is good, then 20,000 is better. The next thing you know, you're up to 40,000, and so on. This is the stuff knee injuries are made of, especially as we get older.

For people who are naturally inclined to be more sedentary, counting steps can be a helpful tool and even inspire them to move more. It's those who take it to the extreme that may need to consider removing the wearable devices or getting professional help to manage their exercise.

When bariatric surgery goes wrong

About eight years ago, I began getting calls from people who had undergone bariatric surgery, and many of them had a shared experience.

The story went like this: They had the surgery, experienced a few months or maybe a year or more when they didn't feel hungry, lost a significant amount of weight, and were able to follow the bariatric diet, but slowly they would start slipping into old behaviors with food and begin gaining the weight back.

By the time they showed up in my office, many had regained all the weight back and more. They had felt too much shame to return to their bariatric team or their doctor. They felt defeated, hopeless, and even desperate. It was heartbreaking.

Through my work with them, I discovered many were overeaters before the surgery; some even had binge eating disorder. Others developed dysfunctional eating patterns triggered by the lifelong diet that had been imposed on them after the surgery.

Many of them who had been using food to cope with unwanted emotions before the surgery were not prepared for a life without their go-to substance. In some cases, these same people would end up turning to alcohol or other substances or seeking comfort through behaviors such as shopping or gambling. I have even seen extreme cases where their weight loss turned into an obsession and they developed full-blown anorexia.

I've seen a host of other issues arise for postsurgical patients.

Adjusting to a smaller body can be extremely challenging for those with a history of trauma or sexual abuse if their larger size had been serving as a protective shield from other potential abusers. For those with overeating issues, mood disorders, or who had been using food to cope with stress, unless they worked on those issues before the surgery, a smaller stomach did not solve their problems but often magnified them.

Fortunately, it is possible to overcome these issues after surgery, but it requires seeking professional help from clinicians who have experience with postbariatric surgery patients.

Reflect:

How many diet programs have you tried? How many times have you lost weight and regained it?

Observe:

How do you feel about letting go of diets and trying a new approach? Notice what emotions (i.e., uneasy, doubtful, fearful, untrusting) and what body sensations you're experiencing (i.e., headache, queasiness in your stomach). Just notice. Don't try to change anything.

Reach:

Allow yourself to be in this uncomfortable place and consider making a commitment to this new approach. Remind yourself that learning something new is not easy but that you've done it before.

But I need these behaviors to feel OK

In order to heal overeating patterns and those companion behaviors, it is important to recognize and honor how they have helped you function. These self-destructive behaviors are in many ways self-preserving. Thinking about them in the context of how they have helped you cope with your life can reduce some of the shame and self-blame.

In some ways, these behaviors have been your trusted companions. They have kept you company and provided an outlet for you. They've helped you avoid painful emotions. They've always been there when you needed them. They have been dependable, loyal, and never abandoned or rejected you.

For the majority of my clients, one of the biggest challenges is letting go of the diet mentality. After about three weeks without dieting, they begin to get frustrated because they are not seeing the weight come off like they would on a diet. They are not getting that ix, that feel-good from seeing the number on the scale go down. They start doubting, get frustrated, and sometimes even become angry with me. I typically tell them I'm glad to see them express their anger since it's a sign they are getting in touch with their true feelings.

Those who stick with this approach will reap the long-term benefits. It is one of my greatest joys to bump into one of these former clients out in the community or to receive a card or email from them saying they are glad they persevered.

The thing about letting go is that it involves a leap of faith, a willingness to believe that if you jump, there will be a net to catch you. It's uncharted territory. Most of you have spent your lives diving into new experiences – college, jobs, relationships, motherhood, and travel – so you already have the skill set.

This leap is like the final frontier. It's the holy grail of leaps. It's going to be scary, but it will be oh, so worth it.

I was always afraid of adventure sports, but in my late 40s I had the chance to go ziplining. The first time I stood on the edge of a canyon in Colorado, I had major butterflies in my stomach. I wasn't sure I could do it and seriously thought about taking the harness off and stepping aside for the next person to go. My guide encouraged me and gave me a gentle nudge. Suddenly I found myself screaming with delight and letting my arms out to the side, soaring over the canyon like a bird. It was exhilarating.

Letting go of behaviors is going to be uncomfortable, but I know you can do it. All the life experiences you've had to this point have prepared you. You may start off flying like a baby bird just leaving the nest. First you hop from branch to branch on the same tree, and then you flap your wings and make it to the next tree. Before you've even realized it, you're soaring through the sky.

It's your time to fly.

SECTION 3: Essential skills and tools

CHAPTER 7: Learning to stop hating your body

The first step toward making any behavioral change is awareness.

By now you have probably gained an understanding of the many factors that have contributed to your behaviors. You probably have also recognized whether you are a stress-sensitive person. What you may not yet realize is that there are three main states of arousal you may find yourself in at any given time depending on your tendency and the situation – overaroused, balanced or calm, or underaroused.

- *Balanced/calm* is the ideal state. It's what you think of when you picture a Zen Buddhist monk sitting in Lotus position chanting "Om." When you're balanced, your entire system functions optimally. You digest food better, think more clearly, and can handle the ups and downs of life. You are neither up nor down but exactly in the middle. You're in the rainbow zone, a place of moderation.

- *Overaroused* essentially means you are in a state of fight, flight, or freeze. Symptoms include anxiety, panic, fear, hypervigilance, pacing, restlessness, agitation, racing heart, rapid breathing, and maybe even feeling like you're choking. Being in an overaroused state can cause disruptions to sleep and indigestion. Some people may even act out in rage or try to run from a situation like a frightened animal.

- *Underaroused* is the opposite of overaroused. This is when you can barely get out of bed, you are tired, shut down, disconnected, or numb. It's like when a bear goes into hibernation and their entire body slows down.

Ironically, when some people become overaroused—overwhelmed by emotions or events – they become exhausted, depressed, flat, or turn to numbing behaviors. They want to sleep all the time, and they may either not want to eat or crave certain foods to help them cope. This is how they run from a situation.

Recognizing our state

Overeating and the companion behaviors we've discussed can quickly bring you from either state of arousal into what seems like the rainbow zone. This type of relief is temporary, though, and you probably feel physically, emotionally, or mentally worse after turning to an unhealthy behavior.

Some people are more prone to a state of overarousal, others to underarousal. Others go from one extreme to the other. The ability to handle stress and how we react in any given situation reflects genetic predisposition, trauma, stress, and epigenetics – what happens to our genes over generations due to trauma and stress.

Instead of seeing these tendencies for what they are, people and society tend to place judgement on themselves or others. How many times have you blamed yourself for being "too much" or for being "lazy?"

With the right tools and a lot of practice, you can learn to live more in the middle, in what I've been calling the rainbow zone, despite your tendencies. The idea is that there is a zone in which our emotions are regulated, and we feel calm and balanced.

In learning to recognize what state we are in at any given time, we can also learn how to give ourselves what we need. For example, if you are in a meeting and start noticing that your heart is racing and you are sweating, you can calm yourself by taking slow deep breaths or rubbing a smooth object like a small stone in your hand.

When we are in the rainbow zone, we are able to be more resilient, able to handle the ups and downs that life throws at us. If you are a stress-sensitive person and/or have experienced adversity through trauma or abuse, you likely have less of an ability to self-regulate when you are exposed to stress, haven't slept well, or are exposed to certain people or situations.

Adverse experiences decrease our resilience, meaning we have less capacity to deal with life's challenges and a greater tendency to become quickly overwhelmed. Learning how to track and shift our state of arousal can be a powerful tool for regulating our entire system.

Finding the rainbow zone

Luckily, there are lots of ways to bring yourself into the rainbow zone. You just have to find what works for you.

For example, if you notice you are in a high-anxiety state before a presentation, you can take deep breaths, sit in a chair with a cup of hot tea, dab some lavender or sweet marjoram on your temples, or all of the above before the meeting. If you feel sluggish one afternoon at work, you can get up and take a short walk in the parking lot, listen to some upbeat music, or do both.

If you notice you are in a state of overarousal – breathing more rapidly, feeling keyed up, pacing, obsessively thinking or worrying about something, or yelling at yourself – here are some simple strategies you can use to calm yourself or bring yourself down to a more regulated state:

- Pet or brush an animal or snuggle up next to them.
- Take a hot shower or bath with lavender salts.
- Seek out soft textures like fuzzy blankets or pillows.

- Use a weighted blanket or weighted lap pad. You can find these online, or you can make your own lap pad by putting uncooked rice inside a small decorative pillow.

- Watch a 10-minute video for yoga nidra, Savasana (Corpse Pose), or any other calming exercise.

- Seek out warmth from a heating pad. This is one of my all-time favorites. I warm up the foot of my bed by placing an electric heating pad down there 10 minutes before I get in. Then I move the pad around to wherever I feel tense or want to be warmed. Don't forget to turn it off before going to sleep.

- Brew a cup of tea and take your time drinking it.

- Find birds or listen to nature sounds on an app. I'm a big fan of opening my window first thing in the morning to listen to the birds.

- Listen to soothing music.

- Take a minute, wherever you are, to plant your feet on the ground and imagine them as tree roots.

- Buy some essential oils, such as lavender, sweet marjoram, or grounding blends. Carry your favorite scent in your purse if you think you might be entering a stress zone, or put them in diffusers around your house or office.

- Create a safe place or spirit place. Seek out a cozy corner or chair in your home. Place meaningful objects you've found, inspirational quotes, or photos nearby. Add an essential oil diffuser or candle.

If you can't get up off the sofa or find yourself struggling to stay awake in a meeting or at your desk in the afternoon, you are likely in a low-energy, low-motivation state. In this case, self-care is about bringing your energy level up.

Try the following:

- Movement of any kind – stand up, stretch, tap your feet on the floor, walk to the bathroom, walk around your office, and go outside for a few minutes.

- Bounce on an exercise ball – that rubber thing you bought for ab strengthening that is lying around in a closet somewhere.

- Play upbeat music and dance if you are able. Yes, you can close the door and do it in your office. I'm a big fan of disco.

- Toss a ball or other object in your hands.

- Use essential oils like peppermint, citrus blends, or eucalyptus that are more enlivening

Managing burnout

Many people don't realize they are burned out until they start having physical symptoms. Physical signs of burnout include:

- Tiring easily
- Sighing
- Shortness of breath
- Chest pain
- Dizziness
- Faintness
- Headaches
- Weakness
- Trembling
- Tingling skin

- Insomnia
- Sweating
- Frequent urination
- Digestive issues

This is your body's way of saying, "Enough!" and "Pay attention!"

If the burnout is related to work, I suggest you talk to your supervisor or someone in human resources. Many companies also have employee assistance programs that offer free counseling.

I can hear you saying, "But I don't have time" or "Maybe after I've wrapped up this next project." Trust me, though, this is not something you want to put off, because it will just get worse. Setting aside time for counseling or taking time off is actually not only good for you, but it shows others it's OK to incorporate self-care into their work lives.

The time for self-care is now. Not next week or next month. Real self-care is about paying attention to what our bodies are telling us and giving them what they need. Treat yourself as you would a friend or colleague. What would you tell them to do?

Now take your own advice. Do it for you this time.

Try this activity to develop some perspective about what constitutes burnout for you and how to address it.

Reflect:

What is your history with burnout? Have you experienced it? When? Related to what circumstances? What was your reaction – that is, did you ignore it and push through, have an emotional breakdown, go numb, eat more, drink more?

Observe:

Looking at your timeline, can you identify any signs that you were heading toward burnout or symptoms you had when you finally hit the wall? Write them down.

Where are you currently when it comes to burnout?

Reach:

If you identify that you are skirting the edge of burnout, start identifying non-essential activities and other things you can eliminate from your life. If you are struggling with this, imagine that you or a loved one have just been diagnosed with cancer and have to see multiple doctors each week. You wouldn't hesitate to drop everything except what is absolutely necessary to make those appointments.

Look back over the tools listed in "Finding the rainbow zone." Which ones would it your specific needs for addressing your burnout symptoms? Use these tools to get back in the rainbow zone rather than living in a state of overarousal or underarousal.

Let's get curious

By now, it's my hope that you understand the importance of getting to the root of why you turn to food and other self-destructive behaviors.

What follows is a powerful tool to help you get a clear picture of what leads to what. This Awareness Tool, as I call it, is a way to gain insight into the correlation between what you have going on internally and externally and how that affects your behaviors with food.

Like many of my clients, you may be thinking, "Oh no, not another food tracking log," and want to skip this section. That kind of reaction makes sense, given your diet history, but I assure you that although this may feel similar, it is very different.

I am not asking you to focus on food or numbers, but instead to hone in on your body sensations, thoughts, and emotions. It will take time to get used to doing this, so try to be patient with yourself.

I recommend using this tool for at least a month to get a good feel for what is triggering your overeating. The idea is to get curious about your behaviors instead of judging them.

If you ate two bowls of ice cream when you only meant to eat one – or none – for example, then you might say to yourself, "I wonder what happened earlier in the day or evening that might have triggered this?" The goal is to become an investigator and develop a deeper understanding of the reasons behind your behaviors.

You can also use this tool for other numbing behaviors. If those other behaviors happen the same time as the overeating, jot them down – if you ate that larger-than-normal portion of ice cream while you were buying clothes or products online that you didn't really need, for instance.

The whole idea behind tracking your behaviors is to educate and empower yourself so you are able to take the steps to change your self-destructive ways.

AWARENESS TOOL

This worksheet is a way for you to gain insight into the correlation between what is going on internally and externally and how that impacts your behaviors with food. It is best if you use this tool daily for at least 3 months.

DATE/ TIME	FOOD & LIQUID	ENVIRONMENT (What happened earlier? Where are you? With whom? What's going on around you?)	FEELINGS AND STRESS LEVEL (0–10) (Note below emotions, body sensations, thoughts, and stress level (from 1 to 10)		
			Before Eating	During Meal/ Snack	After Eating
	i.e., a large bag of chips and 2 glasses of wine	Sitting in front of the TV, alone, in my living room. Had a rough day at work with no break.	i.e., lonely, empty, stress = 9	Numb, calm, stress = 2	Angry with self, hopeless, physically uncomfortable, stress = 9

Once you have used the Awareness Tool, you will begin to see patterns, particularly people, situations, and emotions that trigger your overeating behaviors. In the above example, the next step is to identify those triggering people, situations, and emotions that led to a binge.

Cause, effect, and action

After you've practiced using the Awareness Tool for a week, review it and do the following:

1. Choose one time during the week when you used to turn to food and/or any other unhealthy behavior to cope.

2. Ask yourself: What event or situation prompted that behavior?

3. Put yourself back in that situation and notice what thoughts, emotions, or body sensations you had before turning to that behavior.

4. Think about it: Did you get any short-term relief from the behavior? That is, what function did it serve for you? Did you feel calmer? Did it serve as a distraction? Help you procrastinate?

5. Did any other factors contribute to your using the behavior? That is, were you especially tired? Were you hungry because you skipped a meal?

6. Ask yourself if you feel a need to take any action based on this scenario. For example, do you need to set a boundary with someone and/or forgive yourself?

Once you have completed those steps, consider if there were any alternatives to that unhealthy behavior. Could you have used a coping tool like deep breathing or reaching out to a support person before and/or after a potentially triggering event? Try not to beat yourself up for not using a coping tool. The purpose of this process is to learn how you might do it differently next time you are in this situation.

Continue to go through this process at least once a week with a different trigger. You will begin to develop a repertoire of alternative strategies to overeating. You can keep them in your coping toolbox, write them on sticky notes, or set alerts on your phone if you know you are going to be faced with one of these situations.

What am I really hungry for?

When I review a client's overeating episode with them, instead of asking why they ate an entire bag of chips, I'll ask them to return to the episode and get curious about how they were feeling based on events earlier in the day or something that was about to happen. Then I'll ask them to consider what they were really hungry for in that moment. Were they looking for comfort because they had just had an argument with their partner? Were they seeking stress relief because they had worked a 12-hour day without a break?

More often than not, they can give a fairly immediate answer. It's rare that the episode just came out of nowhere.

Most of us have been conditioned starting in childhood to associate food with comfort.

How many of us can remember being taken out for ice cream or candy after getting a shot at the doctor's office or having our mom hand us warm, gooey chocolate chip cookies when we had a bad day?

Of course, it's perfectly understandable that we turn to food at times for comfort. Problems arise when we do it consistently. This usually indicates we are ignoring our true needs and using food to take care of them.

We convince ourselves that the food is the problem or that it's about a lack of willpower or self-discipline. The cravings actually go much deeper. They represent our unmet needs, our longings for what we are missing in our lives.

The types of food we crave symbolize these deeper unmet needs, and the code for food cravings is actually pretty obvious when you think about it.

How do food cravings relate to emotions?

- You crave ice cream, pudding, or other soft/creamy foods, when you want to be soothed or comforted.

- Chips, crackers, popcorn, or nuts probably mean you want relief from anger, frustration, or irritation.

- If you're craving something warm and gooey like mac and cheese, it's likely connection or nurturing you need.

- If it's a cold, icy, bubbly beverage you want, you may need to wake up, be energized, or find joy.

- If you're reaching for something spicy, then it's likely stimulation or excitement that you actually crave.

- Chocolate cravings often mean you want romance, closeness, or sexual intimacy.

Reflect:

What are your go-to foods? Take a few minutes to journal about these foods and what they mean to you, what purpose they serve when you turn to them.

Observe:

Notice what emotions come up when you think about these foods. Close your eyes and picture these foods. Think about what they smell like, taste like, how they look, and what it feels like to hold them or have them in your mouth. Notice any sounds, like crunching.

Reach:

Set up a place that is calm and neutral and feels safe and try eating a small portion of one of these foods during your daily snack time. Invite a safe and understanding companion to eat with you.

Follow these instructions for a mindful snack: Be sure to give yourself about 15 minutes to eat, and after you've finished, have your companion take the plate away and immediately turn to a distracting activity – plan for this activity just as you planned for the snack. Be sure your companion remains with you for an hour afterward, and don't forget to congratulate yourself for successfully completing this challenge.

The following practice activity can help increase your awareness of the intersection between emotional and physical hunger. You can use it in conjunction with the Awareness Tool.

What am I really hungry for?

Identify a recent time when you turned to food:

_____

_____

What was the preceding event/situation?

_____

_____

What emotions and/or body sensations were you experiencing?

_____

_____

Looking back, what is it you think you actually needed – comfort, support, peace, rest, or something else?

_____

_____

What tools/skills could you have used meet those needs?

_____

_____

Making peace with your body

Thankfully, there's been a slight societal shift that encourages appreciation of all body types.

Some companies are starting to use women of all sizes in their marketing campaign and we are seeing more diversity of body types on TV.

Imagine for a moment that we were all blind. We couldn't see ourselves in the mirror or what anyone else looked like. There would be no fat chat or comparing our size or looks to anyone else's. It's hard to fathom.

We are very much living in a world where bodies are objectified. It's a good sign that there are body-positive pool parties and entire movements to help people feel better about their bodies, but we still have a lot of work to do, primarily because the focus is still on our outer shell, not our internal world.

I am not criticizing the body-positive movement, and if it's working for you, that's wonderful. I've just counseled enough women to know that it's difficult to go from years of hating your body to loving what you see in the mirror. This is why I encourage my clients to start with body neutrality. This means the short-term goal is having neither a negative nor positive stance toward your body; you simply are able to see it and accept it for what it is. Ideally, you will be able to love your body one day but that could take some time.

As you work toward making peace with your body, let's do some digging to gain a better understanding of what specifically in your life led to this war on your body.

Creating a "body timeline"

Before you start this activity, plan to have a couple of coping resources available in case you experience strong emotions, body sensations, or negative thoughts. Choose one tool from your repertoire to either bring you down from a state of overarousal or bring you up from being underaroused. For instance, you might have a weighted lap pad on hand to calm yourself and a bouncy ball to enliven you.

Reflect:

Take some time to consider the messages you've received about your body type and size over your lifetime. It may have been something like "You need to lose weight if you're going to get a boy to like you." These messages could have come from parents, siblings, peers, healthcare providers, teachers, or coaches. Start with your earliest memories and create a timeline.

Observe:

Do you have any memories of liking your body or a time when you didn't really pay much attention to what your body looked like? If not, that's OK. Instead, try to imagine when you were an infant, a time before you had any body awareness other than your immediate needs like hunger, needing a diaper changed, or wanting to be held.

When do you first remember not liking your body? What were the messages you received from family, friends, teachers, medical providers, coaches, and the media about your body, their bodies, and bodies in general?

Think about any activities you were involved in that included your body, like sports, clubs, or dance. Did you have any illnesses or injuries that affected your body in any way?

You can organize this timeline or just write free flow. What have you done to try to change your body over time?

Notice if you experience any emotions, thoughts, or body sensations during or after this activity. Be sure to use one of the strategies we've explored to help you cope with whatever arises.

Reach:

Find a picture of yourself as a baby and put it somewhere you will see it every day – perhaps on your mirror, in the front of your journal, or in the space you created with special items in your home or office. When you look at the photo, remind yourself that you were loveable, that your body was perfect just as it was, and that it is the same body you were born with and it deserves to be treated with kindness. When appropriate, say these things out loud while looking at the photo.

Consider the possibility that your body really isn't the enemy and that it actually may not be that bad. I'm not asking you to love the body that you've hated all these years, just be willing to consider it's not as bad as you've been telling yourself.

If hating on your body is supposed to motivate you to change it, how effective has that been for you? It might temporarily motivate you to start a diet and exercise program, but if this approach worked, you wouldn't still be seeking a solution to your issues with food.

Finding objectivity

For many people body hatred is a way of life.

I've heard women say some nasty things about their bodies. The words they use to describe their bodies are hateful, abusive, judgmental and shaming. It's one of the hardest parts of being a therapist who works in this field.

You may not even be aware of all the ways you've mistreated your body with your words. Let's work on developing a more neutral stance.

Reflect:

Write a list of the negative things you say to yourself about your body

Observe:

Notice any emotions or physical sensations that come up for you as you write this list.

Reach:

Now write down any objective statements you can come up with about the parts of your body that you tend to berate. For example, if you wrote "fat thighs" on your first list, jot down something next to it like, "My thighs help me walk and take me where I need to go."

Practice standing in front of the mirror. When the negative talk starts, respond by acknowledging that you hear it and then tell yourself, "My arms help me hold babies, give hugs, and carry things" or "My stomach digests food so I have the energy to live and breathe."

Post this list on whatever mirror you use on a regular basis. Repeat these objective phrases as you look at yourself. If you don't want to stand in front of the mirror, you can do this same exercise sitting in a chair, in bed, or anywhere you are comfortable.

You may eventually learn to love your body and say positive things about it, but don't put pressure on yourself to be somewhere you aren't.

When you get to the point that you've stopped hating on your body and started appreciating it for what it can do for you, you've reached a milestone in your journey.

Chapter 8: Living in your body

Your body is the source of a lot of wisdom. By listening to it and paying attention to what it is telling you, you are not only honoring this gift, but gaining the knowledge to help you overcome overeating and other attempts to block you from accessing inner peace.

When you struggle with overeating, that's often a sign you are disconnected from your body. Most people have learned to see their bodies as objects and use phrases like "I'm fat" or "I have big thighs" to describe themselves.

Factors that contribute to this person/body separation include:

- High stress levels
- Societal focus on valuing appearance over who you are as a person
- Bullying
- Companies and products that target what's "wrong" with your body
- Weight or size stigma
- Sexual orientation or gender identity discrimination
- Sexual abuse or harassment

In this world of intense focus on our bodies, it's logical that we have taken to objectifying ourselves as a way to cope. Think about the last time you were at a cocktail party or out for dinner with a group of people. How much of the conversation was related to how people looked, what they eat, what exercises they do? All of this objectification results in a culture of constant comparison, causing many of us to come up short and feel shame.

The opposite of disconnection is embodiment – living in your body or living life informed through the senses of the body. It's actually a simple, straightforward concept that involves a skill most of us were born with: connecting with our body sensations.

Simply put, a body sensation refers to your experiences as they relate to your senses such as touch, taste, smell, temperature, or pain.

The idea is that we learn to connect with ourselves through our bodies rather than our heads – that our bodies are the containers for the expression of our entire self and that we can derive great wisdom from paying attention to what our bodies are telling us. It's a primitive concept, one that we have strayed far from in modern society.

Connecting with body sensations

It may take some time to begin noticing what's going on inside your body since you've been cut off from it for so long.

The following cheat sheet can help you identify and put words to your body sensations. Once you become more attuned to those sensations, you will eventually be able to translate them into the language of emotions.

Achy	Airy	Blocked	Breathless	Bruised	Bubbly
Burning	Buzzy	Calm	Clenched	Closed	Cold
Congested	Constricted	Contracted	Cool	Dark	Dense
Disconnected	Dizzy	Draining	Dull	Electric	Empty
Energized	Expanded	Expansive	Floating	Flowing	Fluid
Fluttery	Frozen	Full	Heavy	Hollow	Hot
Icy	Itchy	Knotted	Light	Nauseous	Numb
Open	Pounding	Prickly	Queasy	Radiating	Relaxed
Releasing	Sensitive	Shaky	Shivery	Smooth	Sore
Spacey	Spacious	Streaming	Suffocated	Sweaty	Tender
Tense	Thick	Throbbing	Tight	Tingling	Twitchy
Warm	Wobbly	Wooden			

Checking in with your body

This is a powerful tool to help you become more attuned to your body. Give it a try right now:

Sit back, plant your feet on the ground, and take three deep breaths from your diaphragm. Now do a scan of your entire body, from the top of your head down to your toes. See if you can notice any sensations. It could be a tightness in your forehead or jaws, or that your shoulders are tense, or that your hands feel numb. Now breathe into those places you feel the sensations, focusing on them one at a time. Just allow yourself to experience whatever is there. If all you notice is that your right big toe is tingly, that's OK. There is no right or wrong way to do this.

I suggest you practice this first thing in the morning and last thing at night:

- Check in with your body before you get out of bed. Notice any tightness, tingling, numbness, or heaviness. Take a few minutes to hone in on those places – take three deep breaths, counting to four on the inhale and again counting to four on the exhale. Remind yourself that your body is a precious vessel that helps you carry out the tasks of the day, that it has suffered a lot of abuse – perhaps mainly from you – and that you are going to work on being kinder to it, just for today.

- As you check in with your body before you go to sleep at night, be sure to forgive yourself for any times you yelled at your body or treated it unkindly.

Check in at random times during the day:

What is that feeling in your throat you experience in a meeting with your boss? Get specific. Is it constricted? Try to come up with your own vocabulary for the sensations you experience.

Many of my clients tense their shoulders for most of the day and don't realize they're doing it. Since I typically start my sessions with a body scan, asking them to take a few breaths and notice how they're feeling, they are often surprised to discover they have a lot of sensations that they've been ignoring.

If you have ever attended a yoga class with hip-opening poses, you might have found yourself crying or sighing during Savasana (Resting Pose or Corpse Pose) or later that evening. This makes sense because we store a lot of emotions in our hips, and these emotions are released when we practice opening poses.

Ignoring your body sensations is no different than refusing to use the bathroom when you need to go. It's not healthy and can lead to long-term negative consequences like overeating and other attempts to numb. So, do yourself a favor and start paying attention to what your body is telling you.

Recognizing thoughts and emotions and knowing how to handle them

Simply put, a thought takes place in the brain and an emotion is the result of an intuitive feeling. Most people I have counseled live mostly in their thoughts and are unable to differentiate between a thought and an emotion. For them, the line between thoughts and emotions is blurred.

Typically, when I ask a client how they are feeling, they respond with something like, "I feel like I'm a bad daughter because I didn't call my mother today." This is actually a thought not a feeling. They are thinking they are a bad daughter. The problem is that when we can't differentiate between a thought and a feeling, we run the risk of our thoughts – especially the negative ones – wreaking havoc on our emotional state.

An example: You forgot to call your best friend on her birthday. You immediately think you are a terrible friend. As the day progresses, you think even worse thoughts like "I am a complete loser" or "I'm a worthless human being." By the time you leave the office that evening, your head is so full of negative self-talk that you are overwhelmed to the point of hopelessness. So, you make a beeline for a drive-through and eat a bunch of food in the car as you head home.

What just happened? You forgot to call your friend. You had negative thoughts about yourself. You probably were experiencing an emotion – sadness, regret, and guilt – but you didn't realize it. As the negative thoughts festered in your head, they fueled the emotions. So, what started out as sadness became an overwhelming sense of hopelessness by the end of the day.

The problem isn't that you forgot your friend's birthday; it's that you attached yourself to the thought that you were a bad friend and that extreme negative self-talk ramped up your emotions.

The key to avoiding this type of emotional escalation is to learn to differentiate between a thought and an emotion and then erect a wall between them.

Separating yourself from your thoughts

Thoughts are essentially words in our heads that are strung together in sentences. You might think, for example, "I'm a bad friend." While this may seem like a valid, rational statement at the time, it is just that – a statement, a few words in your head. You can't deny you forgot to call your friend on her birthday, but the problem is you beat yourself up for it.

If you continue down this road of thinking, you are going to feel worse and eventually turn to one of your trusted companions, an unhealthy behavior to cope, but what if you were to look at the thought for what it is? What if you were to say to yourself, "Those are just words in my head" or "I hear you, thought, but I know if I keep listening to you, I'm going to end up at the drive-through. And I don't want to do that today. So, I'm going to acknowledge your presence but not allow you to take over my head." You could even just say, "There's that bad friend thought again."

Essentially, what I'm asking you to do is to start separating yourself from the thought. Imagine the thought is a bully standing in front of you. Chances are you are not going to engage the bully and keep standing there all day. You are going to notice the bully and walk away, choosing a path that will get you where you need to go without getting beaten up.

We can't change the thoughts, but we can choose how we treat them or react to them.

I will often stop clients mid-sentence and ask if they are describing a thought or a feeling. For example, when I ask a client how she felt when her mother yelled at her, she might say, "I felt like I was a bad daughter." I stop her there and ask if that is a thought or a feeling, and most of the time the response is "a feeling." I then explain that the thought – words in her head that have been ingrained for many years – is "I'm a bad daughter," and the feeling is something like sadness or hopelessness or another emotion.

Adhering to these often-distorted thoughts is not helpful, but we also don't want to ignore them. The key is to acknowledge them – "Oh, there's that bad daughter thought again" – and even get curious about them. You may start to wonder why you seem drawn to a particular thought. Is it because your mother constantly reminded you that you were not the daughter she hoped for?

Once this happens, you can find a way to manage the thought better – decide to put it on a leaf in a stream and watch it float away, or say to it, "You are not helping me right now, so I'm going to choose not to listen to you and move on to something else."

Opening up to emotions

An emotion, on the other hand, is like one of our senses – it's important information that is there to tell us something. If we pay attention to our emotions, we learn what we need. If we are sad, we need comfort. If we are fearful, we may need safety.

It's important to pay attention to emotions even if they are painful. It's only when we avoid them that we get into trouble. The longer we try to repress them, the more likely we will turn to an unhealthy behavior to cope.

Once we are more attuned to our body sensations, we are ready to take the next step – giving ourselves permission to connect with our emotional state. As we allow ourselves to experience the full range of our emotions and to understand the unmet needs they are alerting us to, we gain the information we need to develop strategies to meet these needs in healthy ways, rather through self-destructive behaviors.

How we identify or process emotions stems from our childhood experiences, culture, and environment. I've worked with many clients who grew up in families where emotions were simply not allowed unless they were "good" ones like happiness. My mother's family motto, handed down from her grandmother, was the old adage, "If you don't have something nice to say, then don't say anything at all." Needless to say, I had my mouth washed out with soap many times.

How we learn about emotions plays into what we decide to do with them. If we are taught that girls should always be sweet and kind, then we learn to keep our mouths shut even if we feel angry. We become masters at keeping the lid on the pot of boiling water.

Once you have given yourself permission to begin connecting with your body sensations, it's time to start translating them into emotions.

The following is a list of possible emotions you may find yourself experiencing. As above, feel free to add to this list as you become attuned to your unique life experience:

Abandoned	Afraid	Angry	Anxious
Appreciated	Ashamed	Awed	Awkward
Betrayed	Bitter	Bold	Bored
Conflicted	Confused	Content	Courageous
Criticized	Defensive	Degraded	Desperate
Detached	Disappointed	Discouraged	Disgusted
Doubtful	Elated	Embarrassed	Empty
Fearful	Fragile	Free	Frustrated
Grateful	Grieving	Guilty	Happy
Helpless	Hopeless	Hopeful	Hurt
Ignored	Impatient	Inadequate	Incompetent
Invalidated	Invisible	Irritated	Jealous
Less than	Lonely	Loved	Manipulated
Neglected	Overwhelmed	Panicked	Passionate
Powerless	Proud	Rebellious	Regretful
Rejected	Resentful	Respected	Sad
Shocked	Strong	Supported	Suspicious
Threatened	Unappreciated	Unloved	Unworthy
Validated	Vulnerable		

Emotions are like waves in the ocean that crest and fall.

If you choose to stand in front of a wave, you will get knocked down. You may feel scared or anxious, but if you ride the wave, you will be OK. It can be helpful to hold on to an image of seaweed. It never sinks; it just simply floats atop the waves as they rise and fall, and the more you practice allowing yourself to experience your emotions, the more like that seaweed you will become.

Giving ourselves permission to feel our full range of emotions without judging ourselves is an important step in this work. If you've been judging your emotions – the very essence of who you are – it makes perfect sense that you needed to seek comfort from food or those other behaviors.

I'm not saying it's easy to allow yourself to experience your emotions, and I can guarantee you will feel uncomfortable when you first test the waters.

The very act of trying to keep a lid on your emotions is what's been keeping you stuck in a cycle of self-destructive behaviors. It's not until you begin to let go and ride the wave that you will be able to start the process of true recovery.

So, the next time you have a "fat attack," check in with yourself and try to notice any body sensations and emotions you are experiencing. Ask yourself what's really going on. Did you just see a post of a friend on social media who just lost 20 pounds and is showing off her slimmer body? Do you notice a queasy feeling in your stomach? Are you feeling hopeless?

The same thing applies if you go to a social event and become aware you are obsessing over how huge your thighs look in your pants. Check in with yourself. Notice what sensations you're experiencing in your body. What is your emotional state? Do you feel a tightness in your chest?

Again, ask yourself what's really going on. Are you anxious about not knowing the right thing to say and sounding stupid? Ask yourself what you really need. Is it to take a break and walk outside for a few minutes? Or maybe you could use some support. In this case ask a friend to go outside with you or call someone you trust.

Typically, anxiety is related to thoughts about the past or the future. If we spend a lot of time thinking about the past or worrying about what could take place in the future, it makes sense we would be anxious. Try telling yourself "everything in this moment is exactly as it should be."

Reflect:

Is there a recent event that brought up a lot of worry or anxiety for you?

Observe:

Put yourself there again. Notice what emotions and body sensations you are experiencing as you think about the event.

Reach:

Ask yourself what strategies from your coping toolbox you could have used to reduce your anxiety in that situation. Could you have asked your partner or another family member to be your support person while you were there – perhaps someone who could walk around the block with you when you started getting anxious? Consider implementing this strategy the next time you find yourself in a similar situation.

Check in with yourself, like you did when we first discussed body sensations: Sit back in your chair, plant your feet on the floor and place your arms comfortably by your side, close your eyes if that's comfortable for you, and take a few deep breaths from your diaphragm. Start at the top of your head and do a gentle scan of your body moving down your face. Notice any tension around your eyebrows and your jaw. Continue to gently move down your body, paying attention to any places where you feel sensations – maybe it's warmth, tightness, tingling, numbness, or even energized. Notice if there is any color or shape that comes up for you as you pay attention to the sensations. If you have a word that goes with any particular feeling, notice that, too. Then take three deep breaths and gently come back to the room.

This time, write or draw whatever you noticed in your journal, using colors if you have them available. Remember to use a coping tool from your toolbox if you feel either overaroused or underaroused so that you can bring yourself back to a regulated state.

As you become aware of and in touch with your emotions, you may also become aware of those people or environments that tend to bring up certain emotions for you. It's likely these situations have been triggering your emotions for a while, maybe even years.

We started this section on essential skills and tools by recognizing that the first step to making any change is becoming aware. So if you begin to notice that spending time with a friend who constantly talks about her latest diet and how much weight she's lost is triggering something for you, again, try to notice where you're feeling it in your body and what emotions are coming up for you, try to name those emotions, and then journal about the experience or discuss it with a trusted friend or therapist.

The important thing is to express the feeling instead of bottling it up inside.

Chapter 9: Riding the wave

Urges to use overeating behaviors can feel strong, overwhelming, and sometimes compulsive. An urge is an involuntary, natural, or instinctive craving or impulse. We all have them, but some of us are wired to have more intense urges that can overtake us and render us seemingly powerless to fight them off.

But research over the last several years has shown that we can change how our brains are wired. This is referred to as neuroplasticity.

To shift the way impulses are wired into our brains, we need to have an intentional process to create new neural pathways.

The following steps are a powerful way to practice overcoming urges:

1. *Name the urge*: When you find yourself thinking that you need to overeat or indulge in some other unhelpful behavior, or when you find yourself thinking that you should avoid a helpful behavior, say it out loud.

   "I am aware I am having the thought that I'm a bad person and having the urge to eat ice cream to feel better."

   "I am aware that I am avoiding dealing with a stressful situation."

   Once you've done that, remind yourself: "These thoughts and sensations are just my brain responding to triggers. I can survive this wave, and I don't have to act on the urges."

2. *Find the emotions:* Allow yourself to name and observe the wave of the emotion. Say it out loud: "I am aware I am experiencing frustration."

3. *Find the function:* Identify what unmet needs the emotions are alerting you to.

4. *Imagine recovery behaviors:* Visualize how you can act on healthy behaviors. Imagine how these actions would affect you.

For example: I see myself reaching out to a safe support person. I see myself practicing self-care by going to a restorative yoga class or putting on a yoga nidra instructional video. I see myself taking a hot bath with a candle and soft music.

Try this:

Refocus: If the urge continues, focus on something else that requires concentration. Try a crossword puzzle or color a mandala. Go outside and take a mindful walk in nature. Each time you practice a new behavior instead of acting on a self-destructive one, you are will begin to rewire your brain to these new healthy behaviors.

Practice this refocusing skill for 15 minutes.

Mindfulness made simple

Mindfulness is another hot topic these days. Let's be careful not to confuse it with meditation, though. While they are related, they are not the same.

The word "meditation" may conjure images of hours sitting silently in the Lotus position which for many people feels overwhelming. I have heard from countless clients and workshop participants that they cannot meditate or do yoga because they can't stop their brains. That makes perfect sense. It's also the very reason that starting a mindfulness practice is essential.

Like anything else worthwhile, it is going to take a lot of practice. You may never be a meditator, but you can learn to incorporate mindfulness into your daily life.

Below are some suggestions for how you can start.

1. Mindfulness in your morning routine

   Pick an activity that is part of your morning routine, such as brushing your teeth, shaving, making the bed, or taking a shower. When you do it, totally focus your attention on what you're doing: the body movements, the tastes, the textures you feel, the smells, the sights, the sounds, and so on. Notice what's happening with openness and curiosity.

   For example, when you're in the shower, notice the sounds of the water as it sprays out of the nozzle, as it hits your body, and as it gurgles down the drain. Notice the temperature of the water, and the feel of it in your hair, on your shoulders, and running down your legs. Notice the smell of the soap and shampoo, and the feel of them against your skin. Notice how the water droplets look on the walls or shower curtain, and feel the water dripping down your body and the steam rising upward. Notice the movements of your arms as you wash or scrub or shampoo.

   When thoughts arise, acknowledge them, and let them come and go like passing cars. Again and again, you'll get caught up in your thoughts. As soon as you realize this has happened, gently acknowledge it, note what the thought was that distracted you, and bring your attention back to the shower.

2. Mindfulness of household chores

    Pick an activity such as ironing clothes, washing dishes, vacuuming floors – something mundane that you have to do to make your life work – and do it mindfully.

    For example, when ironing clothes, notice the color and shape of the clothing, the patterns made by the creases, and the new pattern as the creases disappear. Listen to the hiss of the steam, the creak of the ironing board, and the faint sound of the iron moving over the material. Notice the grip of your hand on the iron and the movement of your arm and your shoulder.

    Again and again, your attention will wander. Remember, as soon as you realize this has happened, gently acknowledge it, note what distracted you, and bring your attention back to your current activity.

3. Mindfulness of pleasant activities

    Pick an activity you enjoy such as cuddling with a loved one, eating lunch, stroking the cat, playing with the dog, walking in the park, listening to music, or having a soothing hot bath.

    Do this activity mindfully: Engage in it fully, using all five of your senses, and savor every moment. If and when your attention wanders, as soon as you realize it, note what distracted you, and re-engage in whatever you're doing.

Develop an abundance mindset

When I enrolled in a course on book publishing and discovered the entire first segment was on mindset, my instinct was to skip over that part.

After all, my role as a therapist was all about empowering others to recognize their potential and reach for their dreams. I found myself thinking, "This is ridiculous. I don't need anyone else telling me how to do it." The course encouraged me to start daily mindset work that included journaling and meditation. My first thought was, "What a waste of time. This course is not what I thought it would be and I shouldn't have spent the money. I need to get to the writing part."

Then I remembered I had been instructed by the woman who enrolled me in the class to follow the protocol exactly. It was designed this way for a reason. I decided to suck it up and do what they suggested.

One of the recommendations was to write out your dream day five years from now. There's a similar exercise in the groundbreaking classic What Color is Your Parachute? by Richard Nelson Bolles. It's about visualizing exactly how you want to live your life down to the minutest detail. This is a powerful exercise that I highly suggest you try. When you've done it, it's helpful to put it somewhere where you can see it to remind you of your dreams.

The program also recommended you read The Big Leap by Gay Hendricks. I found this book to be full of "aha" moments. Hendricks helps you discover the obstacles that have stood in the way of pursuing your dreams and inspires you to seek the abundant life you deserve.

Something else I started doing was listening to a daily meditation on abundance. There are several on YouTube. Ideally, you'll want to aim for one in the morning and one at night.

Between the meditations, Hendricks' book, spending a lot of time thinking about what I value, and of course meeting with my coach/therapist Gail, I began opening myself up to the idea that I could have my dream life. I also created more places in my home and office with objects that bring me pleasure and offer inspiration. I now have three separate locations filled with these treasures. There's a photo with the quote "Never Give Up" that I bought from a lovely woman on a street in Los Angeles. My intention was to put the photo in my work office for my clients, but I decided I wanted it. It's my motto now.

Developing an abundant mindset involves surrendering the old, letting go of the beliefs that have weighed you down and prevented you from creating a life that aligns with your truest self and innermost desires.

Mindset is not only the foundation of your journey toward healing from overeating; it's also the basis for living the life of your dreams.

All it takes to develop a more abundant mindset is willingness and practice.

If it worked for me, it can work for you, too.

Connecting with your values

One of the biggest challenges of being an eating disorder therapist is that many who come for treatment are not always motivated to change. The behavior has been serving a purpose in their lives – whether it's to cope with anxiety, stress, relationship problems, or trauma – but once we begin focusing on what gives their life meaning and how their restricting or overeating and other unhealthy behaviors are preventing them from living a life they value, I typically see a shift in their attitude.

I once worked with a woman in her late 20s who refused help until I brought her husband in for a session. When he brought up the topic of starting a family, she broke down in tears. I asked her if she wanted to have children and tears welled up in her eyes. This became her motivator. She valued having a family and knew that if she continued her unhealthy eating behaviors, this would never happen. Years later, after she recovered, I found out she was pregnant and smiled inside.

It's hard to feel motivated to change when what you're doing has become familiar and is helping you to cope.

It's like hiking up a mountain, when all you can think about is how hard it is instead of focusing on the gorgeous panoramic view at the top and how good you will feel knowing that you did it. If, as you are sweating and trying to catch your breath, you can keep your focus on the flowers along the way, the sound of the birds, and the goal of getting to the top and seeing that gorgeous view, the pain will still be there, but it will make the climb a little easier.

Likewise, focusing on your values doesn't eliminate the pain, but it does increase your motivation and makes the climb more bearable.

What do I value?

It seems so obvious. We know what's important to us. We are intelligent, capable individuals leading successful lives. Of course, we know what matters.

Understanding what we value is harder than it seems, especially for those of us who have been living in high freeze, going through the motions for years. I didn't realize how much I valued peace and quiet until I started working more from home. It highlighted the fact that I've been living in chaos and noise for most of my adult life. No wonder I was stressed.

Other things I discovered I value:

- Time in nature
- Writing

- The ability to make an impact on a larger community
- Being around other empowered women who aren't afraid to show their vulnerability
- Being authentic
- Spending time with my husband and daughter
- Alone time
- My pets
- Being able to travel to culturally diverse locations

Reflect:

Who/What is on your list of values?

Consider the following: Family, friends, the larger community, health, career, education, leisure activities, religion, spirituality, money, free time, nature, personal style, creativity, time to yourself, music, art, travel.

Who/What do you devote time and energy to that's not on your list of values? Consider why these don't align with your values. What function might these people, things, or activities not aligned with your values be serving?

Let's say, for example, you spend a lot of time shopping for clothes online, but you actually hate shopping and feel anxious about the money you're spending. In thinking about what purpose this is serving, you may realize that it's a form of numbing out from the stress of your chaotic home life.

Observe:

Consider what is keeping you stuck pursuing things you don't value instead of spending time and energy on those things you identified on your list of values.

Reach:

What are some things you could do to move in the direction of who/what is important to you? Develop a plan for how you can start removing some of the barriers to being more aligned with your values, and insert some of those things that are important to you into your life.

Let's try an example.

You are faced with a decision about whether to leave your job. It's a high-paying job with an impressive title, but you are literally expected to work 24/7 because your boss is a workaholic who demands that you work like her. Your family and friends have been complaining that you are usually not around for them and that you are always irritable and angry when you are.

Your coworkers avoid you because you are always angry. You aren't sleeping and you've developed acid reflux.

1. You write down what's important to you and discover that you value having fun with your children, spending time with your husband in the evenings on your patio, and having good relationships with your friends and coworkers.

2. You determine that your job and the amount of time you spend working is getting in the way of what you value most.

3. You figure out that you don't set boundaries with your boss because you are afraid she will get angry and fire you.

4. You could choose to talk to your boss about reducing the amount of time that you work, or you could start looking for a new job with flex time or reduced hours as non-negotiable factors for employment.

Additional strategies

One mistake a lot of new therapists make is to start with a deep dive into a client's emotions and past. In my first year as a therapist, I would think I was doing great work when a client would come unraveled in my office and break down in tears or express deep-seated anger in the first few sessions. What I didn't realize was that they would then feel exposed and vulnerable and have to live with that rawness until I saw them again. They would come back the next week and their behaviors would be worse. Essentially, I had opened up their wounds without giving them any tools to cope with their emotions. No wonder they struggled with stopping their overeating behaviors.

What I've learned since is that the number one priority for helping people overcome overeating is to help them develop alternate ways of coping. It is almost impossible to let go of a behavior that has been serving as a resource without replacing it with one that can fill the void.

Create a coping toolbox

Find a shoebox and use it to create a coping skills box that incorporates the five senses. Include items that smell good, feel good to touch, are pretty to look at and help you feel cared for or inspired. You may even consider collaging the box with pictures you like or inspirational quotes. Many of my clients enjoy decorating the outside (and inside) of their box.

Your toolbox may include:

- A stress ball for squeezing or tossing
- Something soft to hold or touch
- Essential oils

- A photo that inspires you
- Crayons or colored pencils and something to draw on
- Mandalas
- A miniature stuffed animal
- Tea bags

Ideas for grounding yourself

Create an oasis or safe place in your home or office.

Choose a tabletop in your home or office to make a little retreat space for yourself. If you can put a cozy chair next to it, even better. Equip this space with soft fuzzy objects, inspiring quotes or photos, plants, shells, or other meaningful objects you have found. Make sure you inform family and coworkers that this is your space and yours alone.

You can also use:

- Grounding blends
- Hot tea
- Soothing music
- Weighted blankets or weighted lap pads
- Smooth objects to hold
- Bracelets, necklaces, or rings with stones or gems

Restorative yoga and yoga nidra

Restorative yoga is a big name for a very simple practice. In this type of yoga, you hardly move and are mostly lying down on a mat in nonstrenuous poses. Props like pillows, blocks, and blankets are used to support your body. It is a wonderful way to calm your central nervous system and feel more relaxed. Many yoga studios offer these classes in the evenings or on Sunday afternoons.

Yoga nidra is sometimes referred to as yogic sleep. It's a form of meditation performed lying down that's intended to induce a state of total physical, mental and emotional relaxation. Some of the benefits of a regular yoga nidra practice include improved sleep, decreased anxiety and an increased sense of calm, clarity and well-being. I recommend practicing yoga nidra in the evening, particularly if you have had a stressful day.

I am a big fan of online yoga videos, but if you are a beginner, I would highly recommend you take a class to learn how to do the poses correctly. Also, there is something magical about being in a community of people who are seeking calm and relaxation in their lives.

Many yoga studios offer a restorative yoga class and/or yoga nidra. By taking one of these weekly classes, you are sending yourself a clear message that you are worth taking time out to do nothing but rest and that you are making self-care a priority. It also feels really good. I truly find that I get a natural high from participating in a weekly hour-long restorative yoga class.

Keep in mind that if you find it difficult to relax, you may struggle with the first few attempts at slowing down in these classes. That's why they call it "yoga practice." Remind yourself that this is learning a new skill, like learning a language, and treat yourself with kindness when you are lying on the floor with thoughts racing through your mind.

If you are unable to lie down or certain poses are not available to you, this is where a chair comes in handy. There are even chair yoga classes. Remember, this is not a competition and every body is different.

Space to connect with your creative self

Many of my clients insist they are not creative.

Most people tend to associate creativity with being able to draw, paint or make a sculpture. I had that same thought for most of my life. I love art and have always been attracted to artistic people, but I insisted I had no creative abilities.

This is an example of how we attach to a thought and let it guide our behaviors. Some of us got the idea that we weren't artistic in school. Those who produced awe-inspiring artwork were creative, while the rest of us had no talent.

Merriam-Webster's first definition of "creative" is "marked by the ability or power to create." Notice it says nothing about what we create. It could be an idea, a flower bed, a meal, a fun event, an outfit, a hairstyle, or a business.

It's not how perfectly you do it, but how much pleasure you get out of the process. If you are stuck on the end result, then you will miss the joy. I had convinced myself that I wasn't a professional writer, so I couldn't write a book. I initially worried about what my colleagues would think about my book, but then I realized it didn't matter because I've found I enjoy the process.

As soon as I let go of the idea that the book had to be perfect and that I was doing it because it was important to me to share what I know with a larger audience – one of my values – I discovered that I really enjoyed the writing. It's something I can do in peace and quiet, which is another value.

We need space to connect with our creative self – time to just be, to do nothing. By giving yourself the gift of time to just do nothing on a regular basis, you will eventually find your creative self – the part of you that's been hidden away all these years.

If you find that your creative juices flow better in the company of others, then you might consider signing up for a class. If you need accountability, ask a friend to join you. There are one-hour, one-day, or multiple-day classes for just about anything you can imagine – gardening, pottery, cooking, learning about tea, basket weaving, knitting, beading, photography, DIY projects, poetry, and writing.

The art of unplugging

Recently I found myself slipping into the technology abyss.

While writing this book, I began eating most of my lunches alone at home. The next thing I knew, I was breaking out my iPad to keep me company while I ate. First it was just reading the news during breakfast, and then I slipped into the habit of doing a crossword puzzle while I ate.

I was aware of what was happening, but I had no motivation to change my behavior. It was comforting and distracting. I justified it because I was under a lot of stress. I knew deep down inside though that this behavior didn't align with my value of being present and mindful during mealtime. I now recognize that if I am craving that crossword during a meal, then there is an unmet need I am looking to satisfy. My unmet need was my desire to eat with someone else.

I'm not suggesting you abandon all technology but instead to consider your use of it and what purpose it may be serving in your life. For example, if you eat all of your meals in front of the TV, you are likely completely disconnected from experiencing the taste of your food and any awareness of your hunger and fullness levels. You are also missing the opportunity for meaningful communication with anyone who may be with you.

Reflect:

Do a thorough and fearless inventory of your technology use – types, times, and locations. Do you surf social media, for instance, late at night in bed?

Observe:

Consider the reasons you use each type of technology – work, pleasure, distraction, boredom, and procrastination. Consider which of these uses adds to your stress level or decreases your sense of self-worth, such as looking at Facebook and seeing before-and-after weight loss photos. What else might you do instead – deep breathing, for instance, or meeting a friend or calling them on the phone, walking the dog, reading, or cooking a meal?

Reach:

Start considering opportunities to unplug, such as while traveling, during walks in nature, or at mealtime. Practice setting limits with your technology use, just like you would for a child.

Examples of limits include:

- Practice waiting to look at email or social media until after breakfast.
- Try putting your phone down and stop looking at your computer an hour before bedtime, unless you plan to use either for relaxation purposes, such as guided imagery or yoga nidra.
- Hide or unfriend triggering social media friends or sites.
- If wearable fitness devices are triggering negative thoughts, low self-worth or self-destructive behaviors, consider locking them up or even getting rid of them.

Set reasonable goals for yourself. For example, if you have been using technology during every meal, set a goal of reducing your use during three meals the first week and then continue to add more meals each week. If you are craving company during the meal, you can listen to a podcast or call a friend on speaker phone or even video chat them. If you find that music is soothing, then be sure to have some in the background.

This is hard, so it's going to take a lot of practice, but over time you will begin to feel more comfortable and may even find yourself enjoying a peaceful meal without distraction.

CHAPTER 10: Learning to speak your voice

I've found that most of my clients have no idea what healthy communication is. Often, that's because they've simply never been taught or what has been modeled for them was not healthy.

Most people waver between being passive – letting others choose for them – and aggressive, trying to control everyone around them.

Assertiveness is the ideal. That's when we express our emotions and opinions in a way that is direct – for example, saying, "I feel uncomfortable when you walk ahead of me because it feels like I'm not important. I would prefer if you would slow down and walk beside me."

The problem with coming from a passive, passive-aggressive or aggressive stance is that we typically don't get our needs met. If we take an aggressive stance, we end up feeling powerless, ineffective and full of shame, which can often lead to self-destructive coping behaviors.

Passive-aggressive communication is an indirect way of asserting your emotions. Let's say you are angry with your friend for canceling on you at the last minute. Instead of telling her you are angry, the next time you see her you make a snide comment like, "You're such a busy person now, I guess you don't have time for your friends anymore."

If you are passive-aggressive you may procrastinate, resist requests made by others or even pout when things don't go your way. Often people who are passive-aggressive avoid facing problems head on which can lead to feelings of hopelessness and even bodily sensations like headaches or gastrointestinal symptoms.

When you are passive aggressive, it prevents you from truly connecting with yourself and others. If you identify with being passive-aggressive, please don't beat yourself up. It's not your fault. You likely picked up the behavior from someone in your family. The good news is that you can change by becoming more aware of your emotions and developing skills to communicate more directly.

The importance of setting boundaries

Understanding your own personal needs for boundaries and learning how to communicate those needs directly is a critical component of your journey toward overall well-being.

I suggest to clients that they begin by increasing awareness of when their boundaries are violated and practicing how they might have handled such situations differently.

In the early stages of my career, I had a supervisor who taught me this formula. I often share this with my clients:

When you...
I feel...
Because...
What I need from you is...

Being assertive is setting about setting a boundary. You may have been taught that you need to say yes to everything and not make waves, but consider the effect on your stress level when you do that. What you are really doing is constantly saying no to yourself, which ultimately leads to a sense of powerlessness and even resentment.

There are different kinds of boundaries:

- **Closed, rigid**. Picture a brick wall. This is the type of limit that's important to use when someone is abusive to you either physically, mentally, or emotionally or the situation is otherwise toxic.

- **Filtered**. Picture a screen door or water purifier. This is appropriate if the situation or person can be tolerated by allowing some of it/them for a short period of time or with certain parameters. For example, your mother-in-law, who is very controlling, insists she come visit for a week. You could say yes to her but limit the time she stays to three days. And then prepare for the visit by going over what coping tools you will use while she is staying with you.

- **Open boundaries**. Picture an expansive blue sky. This is when you feel safe with a person or situation and you are confident that they/it will not trigger your self-preserving behaviors.

Setting boundaries will likely be uncomfortable, especially at first. Doing so might bring up fear of rejection or abandonment; conflict with what you have always thought to be true – such as putting others' needs in front of yours at all times; or create anxiety about what others think of you, especially that you're being selfish.

Boundary setting is work – hard work – and requires a lot of practice. It's not for the faint of heart but with persistence, you can master it.

Reflect:

Think of a time recently when someone violated your personal boundary. See if you can put yourself back in that situation.

Observe:

Notice any thoughts, emotions, or body sensations that you may have been experiencing. Pay attention to how the old behavior of not setting a boundary may have functioned for you. What purpose has it been serving?

Reach:

Consider what you could have done to set a boundary in that situation. Visualize what that might have looked like. Practice using the assertiveness formula by either writing down or saying out loud or writing down what you could have said. The next time a situation arises, go through the same exercise. You can start by sitting in front of an empty chair and practicing what you would say or how you would act in setting a boundary. Then you can choose a trusted friend or loved one to role play with you, and ask them to provide feedback. When you feel ready to take the plunge, practice setting a boundary with something that seems easier and/or with someone who feels safe to you. Work your way up to setting a boundary with a situation or person who is more challenging. Be sure to process each experience with a support person and/or journal about it.

Practicing setting boundaries is a way to build our sense of self-worth and self-confidence. The journey to building our boundary muscle is like that hike up the mountain. There will be twists and turns, and you may even fall down, but if you keep putting one foot in front of the other, you will make it to the top.

Letting go of the diet mentality

Most of you have been dieting for as long as you can remember. It's been a way of life – a language you learned at likely learned at a young age that is comfortable and predictable.

Letting go of anything that's familiar can be uncomfortable. What makes it particularly hard about relinquishing the diet mentality is that you will be going against the norm.

I have found for many of my clients, letting go of dieting is similar to going through the grief process. At various times they might feel denial, sadness, or anger. I've seen them revert back to dieting in an attempt to avoid dealing with their emotions. I've also heard a lot of them try to negotiate by saying things like "but this new diet is different," or "I don't think your way is going to work for me."

Keep in mind that dieting has likely served multiple purposes in your life so it's important to treat yourself with compassion as you work your way through this process.

Reflect:

What is keeping you from letting go of trying to control your weight with diets? What is your biggest fear? For chronic dieters, often it is never reaching their goal weight, that picture they have in their head of what life would be like if they were thin.

What do you think would happen if you let go?

Observe:

Imagine you are playing tug-of-war with the diet mentality. Your muscles are aching, and you are exhausted from holding on so tightly, but you are determined to win. You don't like the idea of losing because you might feel bad. Your friends – all those diets – are encouraging you to hold on just a little longer. You are worried that if you let go, you will disappoint your "friends" and feel like a failure.

But you let go anyway. Notice what it feels like to stop struggling. You may have a temporary thought that you should have hung on and that you're a loser, but let yourself feel the relief.

You are free of the struggle. You are no longer punishing your body. You can walk away and do something that actually feels good.

Reach:

Create an image of you on a diet. You can either draw it or visualize it. Then journal as if the diets are speaking about their function in your life

Create an image of your true self and choose words to describe that authentic side of you – playful, creative, and adventurous. Use colors that resonate with your true self.

Give yourself permission to let go of the diets. Imagine being surrounded by a circle of glowing light as you welcome your true self into your life.

Overcoming shame

If you're an overeater, chances are you are filled up with shame. Shame is guilt's demonic relative that sets up shop in your brain and shrouds your entire being.

I'll never forget the time in I was in treatment when a therapist covered me from head to toe with a blanket to illustrate how shame had practically suffocated me. Remember, shame is thinking there is something really wrong with you, that you must be crazy for continuing to do what you do, that if anyone knew about your overeating they would be horrified, and that you are ugly and fat. It's a deep-seated, festering sensation that is rotting inside of you and weighing you down, preventing you from any kind of authentic connection with yourself or others.

Shame is feeling bad about who you are. There's a vicious cycle that takes place for overeaters. They overeat because they either have low self-worth and/or they start dieting and keep failing and gain weight (a physical manifestation of their failure) and so the cycle continues. Shame perpetuates these behaviors. It's the fuel that drives them.

Although uncomfortable, recognizing shame and exploring the reasons behind it are an important part of the healing process.

Reflect:

When and how did the cycle of shame begin for you? What messages have you been internalizing about yourself all these years?

Observe:

See if you can notice where you tend to hold that shame in your body. What sensations come up for you? What does it look like? What color is it?

Reach:

Practice the tug-of-war "letting go" exercise with shame.

Keep in mind you've been living with the shame for a long time. As insidious as it is, it's entrenched and it's not going away anytime soon.

The opposite of shame is self-compassion. As you begin to practice regular eating, giving yourself what you need, aligning your life with what truly matters to you, and moving your body in ways that feel good, the shame will have less room to breathe and will eventually suffocate.

CHAPTER 11: Meals, weight, movement, and sleep

Below is my tried-and-true list of do's and don'ts followed by specific suggestions for mealtime strategies, eating alone, eating with others, and incorporating pleasure foods – those foods you've been either overeating or depriving yourself of that you truly enjoy.

The majority of my clients haven't practiced these behaviors since childhood, or maybe ever. While they are simple and logical, it is going to feel like starting over. Remember to be gentle with yourself. I suggest you aim for incorporating one new behavior, master that, and then add another and so on. There's no rush. You've been speaking this other language for years, so it's going to take a lot of practice and time.

Tips to avoid overeating

- Stay consistent. Eat meals and snacks around the same time every day.
- Eat sitting down without distraction at least one meal a day. At this meal, avoid TV, reading, your computer, or your smartphone.
- If you eat quickly, slow it down. Take smaller bites. Put your fork down between bites. Take time to chew.
- If you eat slowly to avoid ending the eating experience, speed it up.
- Set a timer for every 10 minutes to check in with your thoughts and emotions.
- Notice the taste of the food.

- Eat in full view of your partner, family, or colleagues.

- Eat in as calm and nurturing an environment as possible.

- Refrain from eating in the car. Put food in the trunk after grocery shopping.

- Refrain from nibbling when cooking.

- Eat pleasure foods outside of the house. Order a normal portion at a restaurant or café, for instance.

- Incorporate pleasure foods two or three times a week. Give yourself permission to eat them.

- Avoid eating while emotionally charged or stressed – when you are in an anxiety-producing conversation or setting, for instance.

- Eat what you consider a normal portion of what others are eating to avoid feeling deprived. Give yourself permission ahead of the meal to eat whatever it is, and tell yourself this is part of the plan.

- Avoid the weekend or vacation splurge mentality.

- Avoid buffets until they feel safe to you.

- Have someone else plate your food at a buffet or party, and then sit down to eat it.

- Refrain from entering the kitchen immediately after the evening meal.

- Plan ahead for triggering events: Enlist a support person, decide what coping or problem-solving skills you will use, rehearse coping effectively in your mind, have an escape plan, and consider not attending if too risky.

Eat regularly and plan ahead

If eating regularly and planning ahead sounds like a diet, it's anything but.

I am not asking you to count calories, weigh yourself daily, or eliminate foods that you like. When I say plan ahead, I suggest jotting down what you will be eating the night before. I don't mean exact amounts or even specific foods unless you know what they are, or you prefer doing that. Some people feel more comfortable and less stressed having a weekly meal plan with specific foods.

Keep in mind that a portion size is relative to your individual needs. I would suggest consulting with a registered dietician to determine what that is for you. Before you see the dietitian, be sure they do not use a point or calorie counting system and that they use a moderation approach with food.

There are a lot of factors that go into calculating what the right amount of food is for you in a day. Most overeaters I've worked with underestimate what that is and are shocked to find out that they have been consistently eating less than their body needs to function at an optimal level.

It can be challenging to adjust to eating more at mealtime or for a snack, particularly with all the negative talk inside your head or if you are not used to eating normal portions of non-diet food in front of others. It takes time to get used to it.

Fortunately, there are many convenient meal-planning options available:

- Enlist a dietitian who will help you plan your meals.
- Use a local or national food delivery service.
- Look for prepared meals in your grocery store.
- Some restaurants and caterers offer weekly meal pickup or delivery.

Other ideas to make meal-planning easier and even fun:

- Start a meetup group of like-minded people for meal planning and cooking. You could have a cooking party on Sundays to prepare meals for the week.
- Enlist your family to join in on the planning and prepping.
- Try meal swapping with neighbors – just be sure they aren't dieting.

Keep in mind, you aren't going to be able to stick to your plan perfectly. If you are too rigid, you will set yourself up for failure. I would suggest that you stay close to your plan for the first 90 days to give yourself a chance to get accustomed to it. Making your meals and mealtimes a priority is about more than the food. It's a powerful way to put yourself and your basic needs first. My general recommendation is that you keep up the planning for at least a year.

It's also worthwhile to create an eating schedule and stick to it. Have breakfast at 7 a.m., for instance, a snack at 10, lunch at noon, another snack at 3 p.m., and dinner at 6.

Having a regular schedule keeps you from getting too hungry, gives you predictability, and improves your blood sugar stability. Eating regularly also provides you with consistency and takes the guesswork out of when you will feed yourself, and it makes eating, which is a form of self-care, a priority.

By eating consistently throughout the day, you may become more attuned to your actual hunger and fullness. Your hunger hormones will regulate.

Regular eating will also help you structure your day, rather than letting everything else take priority and dictate your schedule.

Once you get used to eating regularly and setting this kind of boundary for yourself, you will find you are less stressed about deciding when to eat.

Mindful eating

If you're reading this book, chances are you are not a mindful eater. Instead, you are likely eating while you type an email, watch TV, or drive to an appointment, completely unaware of the taste of the food you're putting in your mouth or whether you are angry, stressed, or sad.

This type of eating is referred to as mindless eating. It's when you are completely detached from the entire eating experience as if you are on autopilot. Unfortunately, mindless eating has become the norm for most of us, and it's a contributor to overeating and weight gain.

If you're not paying attention to what's going into your mouth, you are more likely to continue eating even if you're not hungry. You are also not getting the satisfaction of experiencing the taste, smell, texture, or feel of the food in your mouth, which leaves you feeling like you've missed something from the eating experience.

Eating mindfully is about bringing all of your senses to the meal. It means you are completely present, sitting down without distraction and noticing what's going on in your body and mind and with your emotions. It's basically a form of meditation, only your eyes are open, and it's done while you are eating.

Meal-time strategies

A mindful meal starts with you sitting down at a table with no electronics and minimal distractions. You are aware of what's going on in your body, how the food tastes, smells, and feels in your mouth. You notice any thoughts going through your head and emotions you might be experiencing. You eat slowly and pause between bites to breathe. You use calming techniques such as soft music or candles to create a peaceful atmosphere.

Practice mindful eating. Set a nice place for yourself and whoever is dining with you. Light a candle and avoid all distractions other than soft music in the background. Try this at least two times a week at first then build up to more mindful meals with the goal of eventually eating the majority of your meals this way.

Other helpful strategies:

- Use the Awareness Tool both before and after the meal.
- Create a calm, soothing environment. Set the table using actual silverware and real plates instead of takeout containers. Light a candle.
- Put on some soothing music. Ditch the electronics.
- Focus on gentle eating and pacing.
- Be sure to have a plan for after you eat. For instance, you can take a hot shower, call a friend, spend time in nature, do a puzzle, or create art – mandalas are great.
- Stay out of the kitchen for an hour after the meal. Ask your partner or a family member to do the dishes.
- If you are eating alone, avoid making extra food. If you do make extra, put it away in serving-size containers before you sit down to eat.
- If you are eating alone, plan ahead for post-meal distracting activities. Be sure to have everything in the kitchen put up before you sit down to eat so that all that is left to do later is wash the dishes.
- Try a bookend approach, such as calling a friend or loved one before and immediately after the meal.

Eating with others

Many of my clients have issues eating with others – even partners/ spouses or close friends. They have so much shame around their bodies and eating behaviors that eating in the company of others can be stressful.

Most overeaters I've counseled think they shouldn't eat anything other than a salad without dressing in the company of others and assume people are thinking "she shouldn't be eating that because she's already fat."

Some overeaters have created a ritual around eating alone. They find comfort in sitting in a certain chair, sofa, or even their bed in front of the TV and surrounded by their favorite foods.

I had a client who ate all of her meals at home in her bedroom. She would place the food on the table for her family and then take her meal on a tray to her room. After using her awareness tool for only a week, she realized that she was so stressed from her work as a hospital nurse that eating alone in her room was how she got a break.

We worked on helping her find other ways to relax including listening to soothing music in the car, taking walks when she came home from work, and sipping on a hot cup of tea in her safe place before dinner.

Eventually, she was able to return to the table to enjoy mealtime with her

She did not think she would be able to do this, as she had been eating this way for more than 10 years, but she did. The first day she accomplished her goal, she showed up in my office beaming with pride and self-confidence.

Practicing moderation with pleasure foods

Yes, you're going to learn to incorporate those pleasure foods into your life and be able to eat them in moderation.

Here's how it works:

- Write a list of those foods you love but tend to overeat. You may want to leave off the foods you find most challenging for the first few months. I had to keep pizza and popcorn off the list for about a year.

- Start each week with a plan for what pleasure foods you will incorporate.

- Try planning to eat two of these foods at two different times during the week. If your choices are chocolate cake and potato chips, then have the cake on Tuesday and the chips on Saturday.

- Plan to eat one serving-size portion of each food out of the house, preferably with a safe person who knows why you are doing this.

- Be sure to keep these and all other tempting foods out of the house until you feel safe around them. This could take months or even a year. It can be especially challenging if you live with others who want these foods around. In that case, I recommend avoiding the kitchen when you might be tempted to go for these foods, such as when you come home from work stressed after a long day, after dinner, or when you're alone. If you know you're going to be home alone with these foods, use your coping tools.

- Keep adding more challenging pleasure foods when you feel you are ready.

- Know that you will overeat these foods at times. This is part of the process. It's to be expected. The key is that you work on changing your mindset from "I've blown it, I may as well keep going" or "I'll just eat everything I can now and starve myself tomorrow." Instead, look at the overeating episode as an opportunity to learn what caused it – say, "I wonder why this happened" instead of "You piece of dirt, I knew you couldn't do this."

The beauty of this approach is that it as you give yourself permission to eat these foods, they will begin to have less power over you. This is how you build real confidence, as opposed to the temporary boost you get from losing weight on a diet.

Reflect:

What are my pleasure foods? Write down a list of those foods you crave.

Observe:

How many of these foods do you actually like? Do you even know? What type of pleasure does each of these foods evoke? For example, if you crave macaroni and cheese, is it because your grandmother – someone who was a safe, nurturing person for you – used to make it for you? Ask yourself if you are getting safety and nurturing anywhere in your life.

Reach:

Look for ways to give yourself pleasure outside of food. Plan to incorporate these activities in your week. For example, if it's a sense of nurturing and comfort you're craving, maybe you can spend quiet time in your favorite cozy chair doing guided imagery, dab some lavender essential oil on your temples, or sip hot tea.

As you begin to incorporate what you really crave, you will likely find that it becomes easier to eat your pleasure foods in moderation. They will not have as much power over you. Then you won't have to plan for them; you will be able to eat them more intuitively.

This process is going to take time, but it will be well worth it.

A note on weighing

There are several camps when it comes to weighing. There's the never-weigh camp, those who weigh daily, weekly, or monthly, and even a smash-the-scale camp.

Ask yourself why you weigh and what purpose it serves in your life. What are the positive and/or negative effects of weighing?

If you decide that keeping track of your weight is helpful or important to you, and you don't react to the number on the scale by beating yourself up or starting a diet the next day, then try the following:

- Only weigh when you are in a calm state of mind
- Prepare yourself for any thoughts or emotions that may come from weighing.
- Plan ahead and commit to using a coping tool in case the number on the scale dysregulates you.

Many of you are familiar with how easy it is to allow the number on the scale to dictate not only your mood but your very self-worth. Weighing is a slippery slope for most people. If you find yourself fixated on weighing and the number on the scale, you may want to see a therapist or registered dietician to discuss how to better manage your relationship with your scale.

Movement

The reason I choose the word "movement" over "exercise" is that a lot of my clients have a distorted relationship with exercise. They tend to exercise for the sole purpose of weight loss or changing their bodies. Exercise for many of them brings up negative feelings and even dread.

Like diets, there are a slew of options for moving your body these days – 24- hour gyms, online workout videos, cycle bars, boot camps, and even treadmill desks. The claim that "sitting is the new smoking" has resulted in a societal fear, almost panic level, that if we aren't in constant motion, we will die early. Recently there have even been studies debunking the theory that sitting is as bad as they originally proposed and instead have found that as long as you get up and move around during the day, you are not harming yourself.[44, 45]

Which brings us back to the topic of stress and how having all this information coming at you has the potential to increase yours. Your stress level may also be impacted by your relationship with the exercise you are doing. For example, if you dread walking on a treadmill in a gym under fluorescent lights surrounded by uber-fit people who look like they've never had a weight problem, this could increase your stress level. Since elevated stress leads to higher cortisol levels, going to the gym could actually be counterproductive if it results in overeating afterwards.

If you aren't stressed by the gym, and it's a sustainable option for you, I'm not suggesting you stop going, but if you hate it and feel miserable the entire time you're there, you may want to consider other alternatives.

Again, it's whatever works for you. It doesn't matter what anyone else is doing. It may be enough that you walk around the parking lot at work while you make phone calls or that you park a distance from the grocery store or take the stairs instead of the elevator.

You may be one of those people who likes turning on your favorite music and dancing in your living room. As long as you're moving your body in a way that feels good to you and supports your overall sense of well-being, that's what counts.

Below are some out-of-the-box ideas for movement:

- Ride your bike around the neighborhood or on a trail.
- Rediscover activities you enjoyed as a child.
- Learn to kayak or canoe.
- Take up water aerobics or water yoga.
- Take up a sport you've always wanted to try like tennis, golf, or softball. Many communities have adult leagues you can join.
- Join a walking club.
- Ask a colleague to have lunch and go for a walk during your lunch break.
- Join a meetup group for hiking, biking or weekend adventuring.
- Walk and shop downtown or at the mall. I refer to these as urban hikes.
- Go to the zoo.
- Take your dog to the park often.
- Sign up for a modern or expressive dance class.

Reflect:

What types of activities did you enjoy as a child? What are some activities you wish you had tried?

Observe:

Visualize yourself doing some of these activities again or trying ones you never did. What are the barriers you might face to doing them? Notice if any thoughts or emotions come up, especially judgment. If you have knee or joint pain related to your weight, for instance, you may be tempted to beat yourself up and think you'll never be able to do any of these things again. Try not to give in to the negative self-talk.

Reach:

I suggest you start either researching how to start one of these activities or incorporating one into your life in the next 2 weeks. It could be as simple as putting on some music and dancing for a few minutes in your living room (if you have knee or joint problems you could dance while seated in a chair). It could take some planning if you decide to sign up for tennis lessons or water aerobics. You might want to inform a trusted friend or loved one of your plan for accountability.

A good night's sleep

It seems society has adopted a policy that sleep is a waste of time. Our obsession with productivity has reduced sleep to an afterthought. At the same time, articles about the importance of a good night's sleep are popping up everywhere, and experts are weighing in on the correlation between disease and lack of sleep.

One of sleep's most important functions is to "solidify and consolidate memories," according to the National Sleep Foundation. Our brains accumulate a vast amount of information – knowledge and experiences – throughout the day, and the cataloging and storing of this information in our long-term memory happens during sleep. "Our bodies all require long periods of sleep in order to restore and rejuvenate, to grow muscle, repair tissue, and synthesize hormones," the foundation states.

Most adults need seven to nine hours of sleep per night; those over 65 need slightly less. And quality matters. If you are in bed awake for several of those seven to nine hours, you aren't getting what you need.

Many of my clients wake up in the middle of the night with a brain full of racing thoughts about the project sitting on their desk, the speech they are working on for an upcoming presentation, or the argument they had with their partner or adult child that evening. I do it, too.

One common piece of advice is to move to another bed or sofa after 15 minutes of tossing and turning. You can also try a relaxing, mindful meditation if you are struggling to turn off your mind or finding it hard to relax.

Signs that you may be sleep-deprived include:

- Daytime fatigue
- Difficulty concentrating
- Less inhibition around food
- Moodiness
- Irritability
- Acting impulsively
- Increased hunger
- Getting sick more often
- Worsening of motor skills, mobility

For overeaters and people who struggle with their weight, it's even worse, as sleep deprivation messes with your hormones. Not getting enough sleep increases ghrelin levels and decreases leptin, which means you are hungry more often and it takes more to feel full.[46]

Some studies have shown that loss of sleep leads to elevated cortisol levels the next evening, which over time can contribute to insulin resistance and ultimately Type 2 diabetes.[47]

Sleep deprivation also causes you to crave the very foods you are trying to limit, particularly the high-fat, sugar-laden stuff. It's easy to see how the combination of changes in hormones and increased impulsivity creates the perfect setup for overeating junk food in the evenings.

Often what I have found with my clients is that the lack of setting boundaries gets in the way of their sleep. They are sitting at their computers late at night either responding to emails or social media messages. They are answering or making phone calls late into the evening or staying up late to unwind since they didn't find the time to do that during the day.

"Sleep hygiene" is a relatively new term for taking better care of yourself when it comes to bedtime practices. You are probably aware of some of the major disruptors to a good night's sleep, which include using technology too close to bedtime, stress, alcohol consumption, caffeine, lack of exercise, or exercise too close to bedtime.

What's important is recognizing that not sleeping enough is not OK and that making sleep a priority is critical for your well-being. If you are consistently getting less than the desired sleep time, I suggest you talk to your doctor about seeing a sleep specialist and/or a therapist who has a specialty in this area.

Sleep apnea

There are also medical reasons why you may not be getting quality sleep. More than 18 million American adults have sleep apnea, a disorder in which a person briefly and repeatedly stops breathing during sleep. In the most common form of sleep apnea, the throat muscles don't keep your airway open, though for some people, it happens when the brain doesn't properly control breathing, according to the National Sleep Foundation.

Sleep apnea doesn't just affect people in larger bodies. You can be underweight and have the condition. Several factors contribute to sleep apnea, including the shape of your jaw, allergies, a deviated septum, and acid reflux, not to mention smoking and drinking alcohol. If untreated, sleep apnea can lead to cardiovascular problems. It can also affect mood and memory.

Symptoms of sleep apnea include:

- Chronic snoring
- Disturbed sleep
- Difficulty concentrating
- Depression
- Irritability
- Falling asleep while at work, doing daily tasks, or driving
- High blood pressure
- Cardiac problems, including arrhythmia, heart attack, or stroke

Some doctors and dentists have started asking patients about sleep as a routine part of their exams. The good news is that sleep studies can now be done in the comfort of your own bed. If you are experiencing any of the above symptoms, talk to your medical provider. There are now many effective ways to treat sleep apnea.

Acid reflux

Acid reflux is "a fairly common condition that occurs when stomach acids and other stomach contents back up into the esophagus," according to Healthline.com. Basically, the food is going in the wrong direction, so it's no surprise that symptoms intensify when you are lying down. You may experience a burning sensation in your throat and chest, the taste of food you've eaten hours earlier in your mouth, and/or a sour liquid in the back of your throat. It can be scary, as you might think you are having a heart attack.

Acid reflux, especially if left untreated, can wake you up in the middle of the night and be a major disruptor to a good night's sleep. Because not everyone who has acid reflux has obvious symptoms, you may have this condition and not know it. If you have disrupted sleep, I recommend you consult your doctor about whether it could be related to reflux.

Some things you can do to help reduce acid reflux:

- Refrain from eating at least two hours before lying down at night.
- Prop your head up on a pillow in bed.
- Avoid spicy foods at night.
- Reduce your stress level.
- Avoid alcohol at night.

Sometimes acid reflux progresses to GERD (gastroesophageal reflux disease). The symptoms are similar, but GERD is when they manifest more than two times a week.

Notable symptoms of GERD include frequent heartburn, difficulty swallowing, coughing, wheezing, and chest pain.

If you find yourself taking antacids on a daily basis, experiencing disrupted sleep, or persistent sore throat, I highly recommend you see your doctor to get tested.

Overeating, mental health issues, and how to manage both

Many people with overeating behaviors also have other mental health issues. In fact, approximately half of patients with binge eating disorder (BED) have a mood disorder, and more than half of people with BED have anxiety disorders.[48]

Some of you may already be seeing a mental health provider for depression, anxiety, or another mood disorder, or you may have been so busy living in high freeze that you haven't realized how bad you feel, taken the time to address the underlying symptoms, or even felt shame for having them. Your overeating may have been helping you keep a lid on mental health issues like depression or anxiety.

If you are on psychotropic medication (i.e., antidepressants), please don't think this book is a replacement for what your healthcare provider has prescribed for you.

As I mentioned earlier in the book, you may experience some intense emotions as you work through this process. Be sure to keep your medical and mental health team informed if your mood or behaviors worsen. You may need more support from them in the form of therapy, adding a medication or changing an existing one.

Please try not to judge yourself. Notice what emotions come up for you and allow yourself to be curious about them rather than judge them. If you had heart disease or cancer, for instance, you would most likely take the medicines prescribed by your doctor.

Mental health deserves the same consideration as any other illness. After all, your brain is an organ just like your heart or lungs, and there is nothing wrong with having to get help to regulate your brain. It is neither bad nor good. It simply is. We cannot change our genetics, but fortunately we can get help from understanding professionals.

Medication

There are a few medications being prescribed specifically to treat binge eating disorder. Your physician or a qualified psychiatrist would know about these. If you feel your doctor or psychiatrist does not have experience treating overeating, you may want to find one who does.

I've had many clients who have been afraid of taking antidepressants or other mood-stabilizing medications over the years, as weight gain is often listed as a side effect. While this can be true in some cases, it does not have to be the reality. Talk to your doctor about your concerns. Since you now know that many factors contribute to weight gain, including unstable moods and stress, I wouldn't throw out the idea of taking a certain medicine if a qualified professional recommended it.

Another common condition that occurs along with binge eating disorder and other overeating behaviors is attention deficit hyperactivity disorder, commonly known as ADHD.

A study by the University of Birmingham School of Psychology in the United Kingdom concluded that core symptoms of ADHD are associated with both binge eating and restrictive eating behaviors.[49]

According to the Mayo Clinic, symptoms of ADHD may include:

- Impulsiveness
- Disorganization and problems prioritizing

- Poor time management skills
- Problems focusing on a task
- Trouble multitasking
- Excessive activity or restlessness
- Poor planning
- Low tolerance for frustration
- Frequent mood swings
- Problems following through and completing tasks
- Hot temper
- Trouble coping with stress

Based on what you've learned about why people overeat, it makes sense that ADHD, especially if left untreated, is a setup for turning to food to find a sense of calm in the storm. My experience with many clients has been that when the ADHD is treated, it becomes easier to create structure and routines with nutrition and exercise.

Know that some ADHD medications can trigger loss of appetite which can be a welcome side effect if you are wanting to lose weight. This is another slippery slope since it could lead to restricting food during the day and bingeing later in the afternoon or evening when the medicine wears off. I am not suggesting that you stop taking any prescribed medication, but inform your doctor, therapist, or dietitian if you are experiencing this side effect.

Another condition for which medication is often prescribed is insomnia. I have seen patients who were prescribed medicines to help them sleep that ended up triggering nighttime overeating. Some would wake up in the middle of the night and, without realizing it, head to the kitchen, prepare food – sometimes even use the stove to cook – and wake up the next morning completely unaware they had done this.

If you are considering taking something to help you sleep, I cannot emphasize enough the importance of seeking out a behavioral health professional with an extensive knowledge of treating overeating.

Finally, a word about diet pills and appetite suppressants: These are typically stimulants. Having counseled many clients who have been prescribed any number of weight loss pills, I have yet to see one who maintained the weight loss for the long term. What I have mostly seen is that these medications resulted in more anxiety and a return to overeating once they stopped taking them.

Many so-called natural remedies include stimulants that can result in agitation, insomnia, and severe anxiety. Sometimes they also include hidden stimulant laxatives, which can lead to dependence. They might also have ingredients that act similarly to caffeine in your body. I strongly recommend that you consult with your physician or pharmacist before taking any of these products.

I suggest you take stock of your caffeine intake too, particularly if you have anxiety or sleep problems. Doing an inventory of all the liquids you consume in a day can be helpful in determining how much caffeine you're taking in.

Fortunately, there are a lot of great teas and coffees that come in decaffeinated versions, so it is easy to find the rainbow zone without sacrificing pleasure.

SECTION 4: Setting up for long-term success

CHAPTER 12: Staying on the path

This is a journey to wholeness, and having a well-thought-out plan for how you are going to stay on the path can be helpful.

While you will never be fully prepared for what life throws your way, it's important to spend some time take working on this section so that you will have a plan for staying on the healing path. You may want to take a photo of this list or download it to your computer or phone, so you always have it nearby.

I suggest that you educate at least one person about what you have learned on your journey so far. Ideally, you want to find a person (or people) you can enlist on a regular basis for the various types of support you have identified you need – the "safe person" identified in the Introduction. Try to identify who that person might be and consider how much you want to share with them.

Some people may not be able to identify anyone they feel comfortable opening up to. They may have scars from being abandoned, abused, or invalidated as children or taken advantage of by those they thought they could trust as adults. If that is the case with you, then try enlisting someone like a spiritual leader, therapist, coach, or other paid professional. It can also be helpful to have different people available to help in different situations – that is, one person might be good at calming you down when you are stressed about how you look in an outfit, but another person might be a great support when you are attending a social event and need someone to plate your food at the buffet.

My safe person or people:

_____

Ways they can help me:

_____

_____

How to enlist your loved ones:

- Encourage those around you to refrain from discussions about weight, size, diet, exercise, calories, food quantity, or "good food" or "bad food."

- Review with them what you learned from this book or have them read the book themselves. You can highlight certain sections for them if that helps.

- Invite them to sessions with your therapist, dietitian, or coach when appropriate.

- Educate them about your triggers and teach them how they can support you at events where you might struggle – social functions, for example, or vacations.

Often loved ones assume that once you have read a book, seen a therapist, or finished a new program that you are healed. Remind them that change is slow, that it is a process, and that slips are normal.

They have probably watched you try many different approaches to curing your weight and body issues, so they may be skeptical, overly involved, completely detached, or even try to sabotage your efforts. You may want to simply say, "I'm trying a completely new approach to my weight and body issues that does not involve dieting. I would appreciate it if you would help support me by reading this book or talking to my therapist/dietitian to learn more about it."

Lapse vs. relapse

A lapse is a momentary return to old and unhelpful behaviors. It's common and normal and is usually triggered by things like stress, intense emotions, or being overly tired. It could be you had a bad day, didn't sleep well, or had a fight with your boss, so you turned to some of your "old friends" for relief.

Another word for a lapse is a "slip." The tendency with a lapse or slip is to assume, "That's it. I've blown it. I may as well keep going (with whatever unhealthy behavior you started). There's no point in stopping now."

A cognitive behavioral therapy term for this kind of black-and-white thinking is "catastrophizing." It's the kind of thinking that leads to increased feelings of despair, hopelessness, and shame.

What if you were to redefine a slip as an opportunity to learn, grow, and stretch?

What would you tell a child, loved one, or coworker if they made a mistake? Most likely, you would say, "You're doing the best you can" or "You're human."

Part of seeing a slip as an opportunity is being able to say those things to yourself.

When you have a slip:

Start over immediately. You haven't "blown it." Yes, you can start with the next meal. For example, if you overate or binged after dinner Monday night after a stressful day at work, start over by eating your planned breakfast at your regularly scheduled time on Tuesday. You may not want to, and your stomach may still be full, but the act of eating breakfast will ensure that you aren't setting yourself up for the restrict/binge cycle to continue full swing on Tuesday.

If you don't believe me, think back to the last time you binged at night and then skipped breakfast and maybe even lunch the next day. My guess is that you ended up overeating that night. Remember, this is not supposed to be comfortable. It does work, though, if you start over immediately every time you overeat. You may not trust this way yet, but you probably agree that the other way definitely keeps you stuck.

Practice radical self-care. Imagine if someone you love had a bad day or got sick, you likely wouldn't punish them or say things like, "You're an awful person" or "You're a failure." You probably also wouldn't lie to them and say, "You're feeling great." Instead, you might say something like, "You have gotten through tough times before, and you will get through this" or "Thinking that you won't get better probably isn't helpful" or even "I know you aren't feeling well, so what do you think might help you feel more comfortable?"

Consider trying some of these tactics with yourself when you have a slip. You might be surprised how easy it is to be kind and forgiving.

If you have overeaten, it can help to do something distracting like a puzzle, pet your dog or cat, or watch a funny movie – you might want to watch something sad that you can relate to, but often doing the opposite can help lift your mood. You might also take a hot shower, do a warm foot soak, or listen to soothing music in comfortable clothes.

Forgive yourself. This is tough when you have just done something that makes you feel worse. Again, practice saying to yourself what you might tell a friend or your child: "It makes sense that you overate because you were stressed," "Beating up on yourself isn't going to make it better," or "I love you no matter what. It doesn't make you a bad person, just human." You can learn to react differently, but it is going to take time to learn how. You might want to look at why this happened. It could indicate you are too stressed and need to slow down.

A relapse is a complete return to the old and unhelpful ways of thinking and behaving that lasts more than a few days and takes hold of you to the point that you don't stop the behaviors. I advise my clients to seek immediate support from a safe person or professional if they haven't gotten back on track within a few days of returning to the overeating behavior.

Lapses don't have to lead to relapses. Remember you can get back on track at the next meal if you use the tools in this book. A lapse does not have to lead to a relapse.

Self-compassion/self-care

By now you have probably identified where you have been lacking when it comes to self-compassion or self-care.

You may not be close to self-love, but by practicing self-compassion by connecting with your authentic needs and desires, the better the chance you will get there eventually.

Things I tend to tell myself or do when I am not acting out of self-compassion or am not tending to my own needs/self-care:

_____

_____

_____

Things I have learned to do for myself (or ask others to do for me) to demonstrate self-compassion/self-care:

_____

_____

_____

_____

Staying in the rainbow zone

It is important that you identify what triggers unregulated mood states so you can create a plan to cope with those people, places, or situations.

People, places, and situations that trigger a change in my moods:

_____

_____

_____

Mood management tools I know to use before, during, or after these situations – for example, deep breathing, asking for support, journaling, mindfulness, yoga, aromatherapy, taking a hot shower, and calling a friend:

_____

_____

_____

Physical activity

I suggest that you come up with a realistic plan for movement that works for you. Consider including activities that you enjoy or might enjoy, such as meeting a friend to go walking in the mornings or after work or joining a tennis league.

Write a list of these activities below along with a timeline of how you can incorporate one or two of them into your life.

_____

_____

_____

_____

_____

_____

_____

How might I include yoga or gentle movement/stretching into my week? Could I schedule and pay for a class in advance, schedule time to do virtual yoga with a friend, or download a yoga app on my phone for traveling?

_____

_____

_____

Nutrition

Remember to be realistic and to forego perfectionism. You don't have to cook a gourmet meal every night.

My plan to manage my meals at home:

_____

_____

_____

_____

Here is where I predict I will have challenges with meal structure – for example, at work, at home by myself, at parties, when I'm traveling, on vacation, or during the weekend:

_____

_____

_____

How I plan to handle these challenges (i.e., have a schedule for the weekend, plan to eat lunch with my coworkers, meet friends for lunch if I'm at home alone during the day):

_____

_____

_____

Sleep

I know that a lack of sleep can trigger overeating and negatively affect my mood. I need to be sure that I get between seven and nine hours of sleep each night.

What are the barriers to getting this much sleep?

_____

_____

_____

What can I do to address these barriers – consult my doctor, re-evaluate my bedtime or morning routine, see if I can start work later, or have my partner make breakfast for the kids?

_____

_____

_____

Stress management

Where I think I will experience the most stress (i.e., during a staff meeting, at a family gathering):

_____

_____

_____

My plan for coping with that stress (i.e., having a coping object like a stress ball or worry beads with me at the meeting):

_____

_____

_____

My plan for reducing stress in my life:

_____

_____

_____

Mindfulness exercises can include a 10-minute morning meditation, a daily mindful walk, a mindful meal, or downloading a mindfulness smartphone app and setting a daily reminder to use it at least five minutes.

My plan for bringing mindfulness into my daily routine:

_____

_____

_____

Body image

Here is when I predict I will struggle with negative thoughts or critical self-talk about my body (i.e., in the morning while I'm getting dressed, when I'm shopping for clothes).

_____

_____

_____

What can I do to help myself during these times? Could I enlist a nonjudgmental friend who is accepting of different body sizes, someone who won't make negative comments?

_____

_____

_____

Social interactions

Examine your level of social engagement. Are you doing more than you are comfortable with on a regular basis? Are you isolating?

What social situations or people trigger my overeating behaviors or negative self-talk?

_____

_____

_____

My plan to handle these situations better:

_____

_____

_____

Don't forget the fun stuff

I recently asked a middle-aged client when was the last time she had fun. She looked at me with a blank expression as she told me she honestly couldn't remember.

How many of you can relate? Maybe you think you were having fun when you took a vacation with your entire extended family, but when you look back on the event, you were actually miserable and stressed.

I realize we can't expect to have nonstop fun, but we can at least try to plug some in a few times a week or maybe even tiny amounts of it daily.

- Turn on your favorite music while cooking dinner, doing chores around the house, or driving. Dance to the beat (or sing and shake your shoulders if you are driving).

- Play with your pets or watch them play. Go to a dog park or cat café if you don't have pets.

- Find a restaurant, bar, or community center that has old-fashioned games like ping pong, pool, or bowling, but don't take yourself seriously.

- Plan nights out with friends regularly.

- Take an art or craft class. Many art studios offer one-time group classes.

- Think of what you loved to do as a child and re-create that experience. If you like horses, sign up for a trail ride.

- Go whitewater rafting, tubing, or even ziplining.

- Watch a funny show or movie, or go to a live comedy show.

Create your list below:

_____

_____

_____

Signs that you are returning to self-preserving behaviors

It is completely normal to experience slips with your thinking and behaviors. A slip does not constitute a relapse. Instead, it serves as a sign that something is off in your life. It can be scary and lead to thoughts like, "I've completely blown it. It is hopeless."

It is important to remind yourself that it is a slip, that slips are normal, and that you are human. There is no way to do this or anything perfectly.

Here are some situations I think could lead to a slip (i.e., lack of sleep, drinking too much alcohol, spending too much time with family, working too many hours, skipping meals):

_____

_____

_____

Here are the signs I am heading for a slip (i.e., increased negative self-talk, eating alone, getting fast food on way home and eating it in the car, stopping physical activity, sleeping too much or too little):

_____

_____

_____

Tips for recovering from a lapse

Practice: Keep practicing the strategies you've learned in this e-book. If you can't remember them, go back to your notes for a refresher. This may be all you need to rekindle your motivation.

Know your triggers: You are less likely to have a lapse when you know what some of your triggers are. Make a list of situations that have triggered a lapse or may do so in the future.

These may include:

- Feeling anxious, stressed, or depressed
- Putting too much on your plate

- Delaying downtime or "me time"
- Being around certain people or places
- Major life changes
- Feeling ill

Create a prevention plan: Once you know your triggers, you can create a plan to better handle those situations.

This plan may include:

- Practicing the relapse prevention strategies you've learned
- Taking some time out for yourself
- Relaxing
- Reading a book
- Calling a supportive friend or family member
- Going shopping
- Trying a new activity for a challenge
- Practicing affirmations

Keep reminding yourself that this is a process. We talked about how this journey was like learning a new language, and you can't learn that – or any valuable new skill – in a few weeks. Give yourself some grace here. You are not a robot. You are a human who is unlearning a lot of old behaviors and practicing new ones.

Ongoing support

A professional coach, registered dietitian, therapist, yoga instructor, or personal trainer can help support you sustain lasting recovery from disordered eating.

Be specific about who these people are and how you plan to use them – for example, see a dietitian once a week, talk to a coach once a week, or attend a certain yoga class on a specific day.

My plan for ongoing support:

_____

_____

_____

You and your support network should watch out for these:

- Denial or justification of behaviors: "I am so busy at work that I don't have time to cook, do yoga or practice mindfulness."
- Canceling appointments with support people more than once. If you cancel two appointments in a row, you are heading down a dangerous path.
- Extreme changes in mood.
- Wanting to spend more time alone.
- Changes in your close relationships.

Identifying opportunities for growth

Use the worksheet below when you decide to try something out of your comfort zone – for instance, when you eat a pleasure food in front of others, set a boundary with your partner or boss, sit in your yard for 10 minutes without your phone, or go to a Zumba class.

Record the situation you are preparing to confront and any anticipated challenges. Write down a safety plan, a backup safety plan, and the date you will give it a try. After you've gone through with it, return to this worksheet and note the outcome.

What situation are you planning as a growth opportunity?

_____

_____

_____

What are your predictable behaviors?

_____

_____

_____

Detail your safety plan. How will you manage this situation? What strategies will you use?

_____

_____

_____

Detail your backup safety plan. If your initial plan doesn't work the way you expect, what alternative strategies will you use?

_____

_____

_____

Outcome

How well did your plan work?

_____

_____

_____

What did you learn from this growth opportunity?

_____

_____

_____

Write a revised plan for next time. Based on your experience, do you need to adjust your plan for the next time you are in this situation? What needs to change?

_____

_____

_____

If you experienced a setback or struggled with this experience, consider the following:

- Setbacks help us learn how to handle things differently next time. I refer to it as "failing forward," using mistakes or failures to make progress.

- Look for nuggets of wisdom in this experience.

- Focus on the process you went through rather than spend too much time and energy on whether you achieved the goal(s).

- Depersonalize the experience by practicing a "growth mindset" rather than a fixed or concrete way of thinking. Instead of thinking, "There's something wrong with me," try telling yourself, "I may need to use a different approach to help me get through the experience next time."

Prepare for holidays, weekends and vacation

Most people I've worked with have the restrict-and-splurge mindset, what I call "vacation mentality." Weekends and holidays are considered times to cheat, and the plan is to get back on track when they return home.

It's a mind game that invariably results in a few days of "being good" upon return, followed by a relapse into old behaviors within a few days.

Stick to the same schedule. Eat all meals and snacks. Focus on the meaning of an event instead of the food. Exercise. Do yoga. Plan for support. It may mean you need to schedule an appointment with your coach, therapist, or registered dietician in the middle of the week or before a particularly triggering event like Thanksgiving dinner or going to the beach in a bathing suit for the first time in years.

Change your mindset and your language. This is especially challenging since most of the world operates with a vacation mentality.

You may find yourself struggling to stay on your path around people who are on diets or who don't have regular eating habits. They may try to sabotage you by pressuring you into aligning with them. This is where assertiveness and boundary setting come in. Remind yourself that it's okay to do what's right for you.

Of course, there is absolutely nothing wrong with eating what you enjoy during the weekends, holidays, and on vacation. What's important is eliminating the all-or-nothing thinking, avoiding the terms "good" and "bad," "cheat" or "splurge." If you are to the point where you can schedule eating pleasure foods once or twice a week, just be sure those times coincide with your weekend getaway or holiday get-together. Planning can help you avoid the restrict-and-splurge mentality.

Remind yourself that this is for the long haul and that moderation is the goal. It will be uncomfortable at first, but eventually you will settle into it and it will become normal for you.

Keep HALTS in mind

While working with alcoholics many years ago, I came across the acronym HALT, which stands for hungry, angry, lonely, and tired. I've added an "S" to create HALTS – hungry, angry, lonely, tired, and stressed. I have found this acronym useful myself and have introduced it to most of my clients. Each one of these five conditions, if not addressed within a reasonable amount of time, leaves you vulnerable to a slip.

It can be helpful to be aware of HALTS. Write it on a card and post it in your home or office. If you don't want anyone to see it, snap a photo and use that as a screensaver.

If you are serious about staying on course, you will need to do everything in your power to make this new way of living your top priority, especially for the first year.

Redefining change

Because change involves confronting the unfamiliar and the uncomfortable, it is by no means, easy, but it is completely doable, especially if you have gotten to this point in the book. By doing so, you have demonstrated a willingness and ability to persevere.

I tell my clients the main ingredient for change is a seed of willingness and the ability to put one foot in front of the other and keep going. You are capable of doing this, since you've done it in every other aspect of your life.

Let's put that ability to plow through any situation to good use now.

Helpful considerations for long-term change:

- Beware of setting lofty, unattainable goals.
- Allow the healing process to unfold slow and steady. You are in this for the long haul.
- Focus on progress, not perfection.
- Recognize any change – fewer binge episodes, eating less than you used to at a party, reduction in negative self-talk, and increased self-care.
- See setbacks as opportunities to learn and grow.
- Replace judgment with curiosity: "I wonder why I am doing this" or "What can I learn from this" instead of "What are you doing, you idiot?"
- Practice willingness or "the willingness to be willing" – being open to doing something differently, taking an uncharted path and experiencing those emotions you've been avoiding, and asking for and being willing to receive support.

CHAPTER 13: Thawing and thriving

There is a lot of buzz about self-care these days. It seems that everywhere you turn, there's another product or service promising to heal you. The fact that there are so many options can be overwhelming.

Most of us get so caught up in the urgency to take better care of ourselves that we don't see what is immediately available to us – walking in our backyard, relaxing in our bathtub, eating a simple home-cooked meal at a table we set, sitting by the fire with a hot cup of tea, or cuddling with our pet. The challenge is that since you probably are of the mindset that you need a product or program to help you feel better, the idea of slowing down enough to use what's right in front of you may feel daunting.

The beauty of the breath

When I meet with a client for the first time and ask them to take a deep breath, it's rare that they know how to do it.

Invariably, I watch as their chest expands, and they take a shallow breath. How would they know what constitutes an actual deep breath if they haven't been taught?

So, I teach my clients how to take deep belly breaths. I have them sit in a comfortable position and ask them to imagine they are blowing up a balloon from their diaphragm. Then I ask them to practice at home while lying down with a piece of paper on their belly. When the paper moves up and down, they've succeeded.

There are a number of online videos and other resources to help you practice this type of breathing.

Notice I said "practice." It takes time to switch from chest breathing to breathing from your diaphragm.

The beauty of deep breathing is that once you have it down, you can use it anywhere – in the car at a stoplight, in a waiting room, in bed, at the table before, during or after you eat, or even in a meeting.

Let it flow: Journaling

Journaling is a powerful and simple tool that has several benefits:

- It encourages you to slow down for a few minutes.
- It increases self-awareness.
- It enhances mindfulness.
- It releases blocked emotions.
- It helps create focus.
- It connects your inner and outer worlds.

I recommend a free-flow method of writing, which means you simply sit down and start writing whatever comes up for you. It could even be just writing that you are tired and don't feel like journaling.

If you are wanting to connect with your inner child – that part of you that is not self-conscious and can express your true feelings – then I suggest you try writing with your nondominant hand. You will be amazed at the rawness of the feelings that come out – just be prepared for some major "ahas" and maybe even some tears.

I suggest you write for at least five minutes and try not to pick up your pen from the paper. It doesn't matter what you write; just keep it flowing.

I know this is a tall order for some of you perfectionists, but I recommend you make a valiant attempt to suspend all judgement about how or what you are writing. Remember, this is not a graded exam. In fact, you can even choose to shred your journal.

So, let go of all your worries about punctuation or how neat your handwriting is. The point is to clear the clutter in your head so you can be in touch with what's really going on inside and feel more centered.

I also suggest that you journal when it works best for you. In other words, there is no perfect time. I prefer late evening, but sometimes find myself writing in the spur of the moment during the day when I feel a pressing need to get something out of my system.

For those of you who are adamant about not wanting to write, you could try five minutes of free flow talking into a recorder or video camera on your smartphone. It's whatever works for you.

Give yoga a chance

I remember trying my first yoga class back in my mid-20s. I had several friends who had encouraged me, though I resisted. At the time, I was obsessed with aerobics and running and refused to "waste time" sitting or lying down for an hour when I could be burning calories and flattening my abs. As expected, I hated every minute of it. It was the opposite of relaxing for me, as my mind raced with thoughts of everything else I could have or should have been doing while I was lying there in Savasana (Resting Pose).

I didn't try it again until I was 44 and going through perimenopause. Desperate to find some relief from hot flashes and mood dysregulation, I read that yoga was beneficial for hormonal balance, so off I went to a yoga studio.

The first class brought up all of my insecurities. I could not do any of the balance poses and my perfectionism kicked in to shame me, and of course, I was comparing myself to all the others in the room who seemed to be able to find balance flawlessly.

Fortunately, the teacher reminded us that it was a process and that letting go of perfection and being patient with ourselves was part of the learning curve. So, I did my Tree Pose with one foot on the ground and the other resting on my ankle for months. One day I finally did it.

Ta-da. I realized that finding balance had less to do with being good at yoga and was more about mindset, patience, breathing, and keeping my gaze on a point on the floor in front of me.

I have found yoga to be a wonderful way to connect with my body, practice humility, and gain confidence.

Unstructured time

Most people I counsel have no clue how to just be.

The mere thought of having nothing to do can be overwhelming. What's ironic is how often we talk about needing time to ourselves, yet when it comes down to actually taking it, we avoid it or feel unsettled about it. We are afraid of what will happen – that we will connect with a part of ourselves that we haven't known for a long time, that we might be overcome with emotions, lose control, or not be able to cope.

I counseled a client who had a stack of massage gift certificates given to her by friends and family over the years. She was a brilliant woman who was highly accomplished in her career. Like many of my clients, her life seemed picture perfect on the outside, but what others couldn't see was her struggle with binge eating.

Every time I brought up the massage gift certificates, she would get defensive and explain she was too busy to redeem them. After working with her for several months, the reason she refused the massages became clear: She was afraid of what would happen if she allowed herself to have nothing to do for an hour. The mere thought of lying on a table gave her severe anxiety. We had to spend several sessions working up to even scheduling a massage.

The first massage was challenging, but the more she went, the easier it became. Eventually she started scheduling massages each week.

The massages became the gateway to an entire new way of life. She began to cut back on her work hours and devote more time to self-care and pleasurable activities – more time for herself. The more she practiced self-care, the less frequent the binges until eventually she stopped entirely.

I had a therapist in my 20s who gave me the toughest homework ever. My assignment was to go home and stay in my house the entire weekend and disconnect from everyone.

I remember the panicky feeling I had the first few hours I spent alone in my house with no plan. The first day was the hardest. I had to teach myself how to do nothing without turning to food. After a few weeks of practice, I began looking forward to spending time by myself. I started to enjoy having no one else to be accountable to and no schedule to follow. I began feeling calmer and more rested when I returned to work on Mondays. I definitely spent a lot of time crying, but they were tears of relief, of feeling more connected to the child within me – to the real me.

I'm not suggesting that you go from one extreme of taking no time for yourself to going an entire weekend. Start with baby steps – maybe take a few minutes a few times a day, just you, no distractions. Then work yourself up to longer periods. As hard as it is to imagine, one day it will come naturally, and you will find yourself craving time alone.

Niksen is a term the Dutch use for doing nothing. It's not mindfulness or meditation. It's just doing nothing – consciously choosing to sit on the couch, in your favorite chair, or on an airplane and just stare out the window.

I do this a lot. No phone. No iPad. No computer screen. Just sitting. Pretty much anywhere I go.

No one else even notices since they are all staring at their screens. In today's society, it might be considered lazy or being a couch potato, but I suggest we reframe the conversation and refer to it as "restorative time" or "healing time."

We all are familiar with the term "hang out." Niksen is just that. We can either hang out alone or with someone else. My husband and I hang out in our yard when the weather is warm. We spend a lot of time talking, but we also take moments of silence to just be in nature, listen to the birds, or watch our dogs frolic in the yard.

Since when did daydreaming get such a bad rap? Sitting and staring and just letting your mind wander – on your surroundings, your hopes and dreams, your family and friends, anything you value. Twenty-first century demands have essentially decimated this lost art. Just imagine if we had daydreaming courses in school or if we had daydreaming breaks at work – time to mentally regroup and reflect and just be.

Honor the art of rest

If you are doing nothing, honor it. Don't apologize.

When someone asks me what I did over the weekend, I may tell them, "I rested" or "I really did nothing." By responding this way, I own my behavior. I'm also indirectly giving others permission to do the same.

People make a lot of assumptions about others' schedules – that successful women are always busy, for instance. What if we were to turn the tables and start celebrating each other's quest for restorative time? It is up to each of us to own this movement.

Think of doing nothing as another life skill that is going to take practice. It will most likely be uncomfortable at first, and you might even feel guilty. Remember, that feeling is legitimate, but the thoughts that you attach to it like "I should be doing..." or "I'm lazy if I'm not doing anything" are when things become problematic.

Setting aside time to rest and restore is the ultimate form of self-care. You'll find that allowing yourself this mental "breathing room" will open up your creative pathways and lead you to your innermost desires. Who knows, you may even decide to write your own e-book.

Try this:

Create "do nothing" spaces in your home or office, spaces you go to without your smartphone or tablet. Set a timer and start small – say five minutes – and work yourself up to longer. Enlist a friend, coworker, or partner to do nothing with you, or invite a group of friends to spend part of your time together doing nothing. Be sure to take time afterward to process the experience, either with the other party or in a journal.

Developing compassion for our imperfections

Wabi-sabi is an ancient Japanese philosophy that focuses on accepting the imperfect and transient nature of life. It's rooted in Buddhism and arose from tea ceremonies in which prized utensils were handmade, irregular, and imperfect.

We waste so much of our time and energy on and trying to mask our imperfections – researching and spending money on products to mask our so-called flaws. The pursuit of perfection is a draining occupation and stress-inducing – and yet another way for us to avoid our emotions. We have built up a mountain of fears about what it would be like to show our true selves to the world.

What if instead of focusing on ridding ourselves of our perceived flaws, we made an effort to get to know them? I'm not saying you have to love your wrinkles, gray hair, or the extra layer of fat on your belly, but is yelling at those things really doing you any good, especially now that you know how damaging stress is to your health?

What if instead of Botox parties, we had "conscious aging" get-togethers where we talked about our emotions instead of how to change our bodies? I read a news article recently about a mother who had a party for her daughter to celebrate menstruation. Imagine if we lived in a world where we celebrated our uniqueness instead of constantly focusing on trying to look like everyone else. What an amazing gift we would be giving our children and those in our circle of influence.

Living to your potential

Trust me when I say your dream life awaits you. Your time is now. If you've been telling yourself it's not possible for you or it's late to change, that's just a barrier you've erected in your head – a string of words that have become a mantra.

You are going to start with developing curiosity about what you are doing and why you've been doing it. Then you're going to begin taking baby steps toward change. As you practice the tools in this book, you will gain confidence in yourself and start believing that you can have a better life. You are going to keep putting one foot in front of another, stay on the path and watch as your self-preserving behaviors disappear and are replaced with real self-care. You will learn that making yourself vulnerable and opening up to others about your struggles will not only empower you but ground you with a sense of connectedness. Along the way you will develop patience and compassion for yourself. You will stop berating yourself and start believing that maybe, just maybe, you are OK and deserve to have the life of your dreams. I believe in you.

Reflect:

What is your dream life? Dig deep. Fantasize.

Observe:

What is holding you back from living that life? What is the effect of not giving yourself what you want – on yourself, on your behaviors, on others? What are some things you want that you don't allow yourself?

Reach:

Write out your ideal day five years from now. Then 10 years.

And then start adding some of the components of your ideal day into your current life.

Part of my dream life is that I'll spend more time at the beach. I recently attended a conference in Charleston, South Carolina. At the end of the first day, we were given a simple homework assignment: do one out-of-the-box thing before we came back in the morning.

My first thought was to show up the next day without any makeup, which I ended up doing, but as I was setting my alarm for the morning, I decided to wake up an hour earlier and drive to the beach to see the sunrise.

I constantly complain that I never go to the beach – beach time is now on my dream list – so I got up and took myself to Sullivan's Island, the beach of my childhood. As I crossed the drawbridge to the island, I felt my body breathe and expand. Then as I walked along the worn wooden path lined with sea oats to the beach, my free-spirited 5-year-old self sprang to life.

Watching the sunrise over the Atlantic Ocean set me afire. I found myself swirling around in circles and smiling. I found a beautiful sand dollar – it wasn't alive – and a few shells that morning, which I ended up putting in my spirit place next to my bed and in my office.

That was my reminder of my dream. I hope this e-book encourages you to make one bold move to connect with what sparks a flame inside of you and brings you closer to the life of your dreams.

Reflect:

When is the last time you did something completely out of your routine, something just for you? What is something you could do that would be just for you, something you have never done or have wanted to do for a while?

Observe:

Notice any emotions or sensations that come up for you as you think about this thing. Are you struggling to come up with something?

Reach:

Do one bold move tomorrow. Keep it simple. Plan it. Tell someone you're going to do it. Do it. Write about your experience. Then keep doing it. Add more bold moves.

Lessons from my yard

I'm a city girl at heart. I love the excitement and energy I get when I'm immersed in the sounds, colors, smells – all the aromas from the different foods – and chaos of the city.

But I've discovered the true peace that for me only comes with being surrounded by nature.

Trust me, I never imagined I'd become a bird watcher. The only birds in my childhood repertoire were pigeons, and although I spent a lot of time in Central Park, I didn't even notice the other birds or wildlife, but today, we have a bird feeder and two suet cages by our outdoor dining table, and one of my greatest joys is watching the birds flocking around it. Now I can identify bluebirds, red-tailed hawks, woodpeckers, house inches, brown thrashers, chickadees, and cardinals. I know them by their sounds now too.

I have literally become obsessed with making sure they have enough food and water – yes, I refill their bird bath every day. I've even rescued a hummingbird and a baby bluebird, held them in the palm of my hand, and comforted them. The ones that didn't make it are buried in a makeshift pet graveyard located under a camellia bush in my front yard.

I didn't start out knowing their names. I just took the time to notice them. Eventually I got curious, and when my aunt gave me a book on birds, I started learning some of their names. Thanks to that book, I can differentiate the males from the females of each bird type, and it all started by making a simple change in my life.

At my last job, I began a routine of going outside and taking mindful walks in the parking lot as a way to center myself. I noticed some hawks flying above me when I parked my car in the morning. Then one day I looked up and saw they had built a nest in the cellphone tower next to our office. Soon after, I noticed there were baby hawks, and I watched how the babies would start out in the world by going short distances to the closest trees and flapping their wings a lot. Then I noticed the babies were able to soar high in the sky.

Since my office had big windows, I started working at a table facing the parking lot so I could watch the hawks as they soared above me. I started pointing them out to clients and my staff. Now I know the sound a hawk makes, and I know when one is around so I can look up in the sky and spot it.

From the moment I experienced seeing that first hawk, birds have become a coping resource for me. The beauty is that they are almost everywhere I go, always available, steady, and constant companions who can fill my senses in a matter of moments. It's that simple.

This is my hope for you. That you will take the wisdom and tools provided for you and start the journey toward your dream life. That you will put up a bird feeder – or whatever your equivalent may be – that fills you up with joy. That you will find the abundance that you deserve. That your spirit will soar.

Acknowledgments

Being able to write this book was a gift. The only reason the book exists is that I was fortunate to have had the experience of sitting across from so many people who were willing to share their struggles with me. This book is dedicated to all of you.

I want to thank my right hand for the past several years Tristan Ramsey for her hard work and dedication and Katie Wargo, LPC, CEDS, for her assistance with research and citations.

Then there are the women in my life who have supported me during a time of major transition: Anna, Gail, Heidi, Lynn, Lee, Lydia, and Sue. You have not only kept me afloat but empowered me to reach my fullest potential. Thank you for shining your light on me no matter what!

Owen, my husband of 25 years, is my rock. He is always here to pick me up when I fall and to encourage me to keep putting one foot in front of the other.

Lastly, I want to dedicate this book to my daughter Clara. Her willingness to travel the path of authenticity warms my heart and is a constant source of inspiration.

Contact

https://rileywellnessgroup.com

If you found this book helpful, please see below:

To help others find this book more easily, please review the book on Amazon. It only takes a couple of minutes but makes a big difference in getting the book into the hands of those who could benefit from reading it.

I appreciate you.

References

[1] Smolak, L. (2011). Body image development in childhood. In T. Cash & L. Smolak (Eds.), Body Image: A Handbook of Science, Practice, and Prevention (2nd ed.). New York: Guilford.

[2] Martin, J. B. (2010). The development of ideal body image perceptions in the United States. Nutrition Today, 45(3), 98-100. Retrieved from nursingcenter.com/pdf.asp?AID=1023485

[3] Andreyeva, T., Puhl, R. M., & Brownell, K. D. (2008). Changes in perceived weight discrimination among Americans 1995–1996 through 2004–2006. Obesity, 16, 1129–1134. doi:10.1038/oby.2008.35

[4] Hayes, S. & Tantleff-Dunn, S. (2010). Am I too fat to be a princess? Examining the effects of popular children's media on young girls' body image. British Journal of Developmental Psychology, 28(2), 413–426.

[5] Dohnt, H. K. & Tiggemann, M. (2004). Development of perceived body size and dieting awareness in young girls. Perceptual and Motor Skills, 99(3, Part 1), 790–792.y

[6] Dohnt, H. K. & Tiggemann, M. (2006). Body image concerns in young girls: The role of peers and media prior to adolescence. Journal of Youth and Adolescence, 35(2), 135–145.

[7] Lowes, J. & Tiggemann, M. (2003). Body dissatisfaction, dieting awareness and the impact of parental influence in young children. The British Psychological Society, 8, 135–147.

[8] Zhao Y. & Encinosa W. (2011). An update on hospitalizations for eating disorders, 1999 to 2009: Statistical brief #120. 2011 Sep. In: Healthcare Cost and Utilization Project (HCUP) Statistical Briefs [Internet]. Rockville (MD): Agency for Healthcare Research and Quality (US); 2006 Feb-. Available from: https:/ www.ncbi. nlm.nih.gov/books/NBK65135/.

[9] IQVIA Institute for Human Data Science, November 2017. Report: The growing value of digital health.

[10] Simpson, C. & Mazzeo, S. (2017). Calorie counting and fitness tracking technology: Associations with eating disorder symptomology. Eating behaviors, 26.

[11] Covey, S. R. (1989). The seven habits of highly effective people: Restoring the character ethic. New York: Simon and Schuster.

[12] The National Center on Addiction and Substance Abuse (CASA) at Columbia University. (2003). Food for thought: Substance abuse and eating disorders. The National Center on Addiction and Substance Abuse (CASA) Columbia University, New York.

[13] Grilo C.M., Sinha R., O., & Malley, S.S. (2002). Eating disorders and alcohol use disorders. Alcohol Research and Health, 26, 151-160.

[14] Wang, G. J., Volkow, N. D., Logan, J., Pappas, N. R., Wong, C. T., Zhu, W., Netusil, N., & Fowler, J.S. (2001). Brain dopamine and obesity. Lancet, 357, 354–357. 10.1016/S0140-6736(00)03643-6

[15] Davis, C., Levitan, R. D., Yilmaz, Z., Kaplan, A. S., Carter, J. C., Kennedy, J. L. (2012). Binge eating disorder and the dopamine D2 receptor: Genotypes and sub-phenotypes. Progress in Neuro-Psychopharmacology and Biological Psychiatry, 38(2), 328-335. doi: 10.1016/j.pnpbp.2012.05.002

16 Broft, A., Shingleton, R., Kaufman, J., Liu, F., Kumar, D., Slifstein, M., & Walsh, B. T. (2012). Striatal dopamine in bulimia nervosa: A pet imaging study. International Journal of Eating Disorders, 45(5), 648-656. doi: 10.1002/eat.20984

17 Putterman, E. & Linden, W. (2006). Cognitive dietary restraint and cortisol: Importance of pervasive concerns with appearance. Appetite, 47(1), 64-76.

18 Creswell, J.D., Pacilio, L.E., Denson, T.F., & Satyshur, M. (2013). The effect of a primary sexual reward manipulation on cortisol responses to psychosocial stress in men. Psychosomatic Medicine, 74(4): 397-403. doi: 10.1097/PSY.0b013e31828c4524

19 Oswald, W.D., Gunzelmann, T., Rupprecht, R., & Hagen, B. (2006). Differential effects of single versus combined cognitive and physical training with older adults: the SimA study in a 5-year perspective. European Journal of Ageing, 3: 179. https:/doi.org/10.1007/s10433-006-0035-z

20 Ahmadzadeh, A., Barnes, M.A., Gwazdauskas, F.C., & Akers, R.M. (2006). Dopamine antagonist alters serum cortisol and prolactin secretion in lactating Holstein cows. Journal of Dairy Science, 89(6), 2051-5.

21 Mastorakos, G., Pavlatou, M., Diamanti-Kandarakis, E., Chrousos, G.P. (2005). Exercise and the stress system. Hormones, 4(2): 73-89.

22 Polycystic Ovary Syndrome. (April 1, 2019). Retrieved from https:/www.womenshealth.gov/a-z-topics/polycystic-ovary-syndrome

23 Parker, M. R., Feng, D., Chamuris, B., Margolskee, R. F. (2014). Expression and nuclear translocation of glucocorticoid receptors in type 2 taste receptor cells. Neuroscience Letters, 571, 72-77.

[24] Kessler, D. (2009). The end of overeating: Taking control of the insatiable American appetite. New York: Rodale.

[25] Austin, S. & Bryn, S. (2004). Sexual orientation, weight concerns, and eating- disordered behaviors in adolescent girls and boys. Journal of the American Academy of Child & Adolescent Psychiatry, 43(9), 1115-23.

[26] Carlat, D.J., Camargo, C.A., & Herzog, D.B. (1991). Eating disorders in males: a report of 135 patients. American Journal of Psychiatry, 148, 1991.

[27] Ray, N. (2006). Lesbian, gay, bisexual and transgender youth: An epidemic of homelessness. New York: National Gay and Lesbian Task Force Policy Institute and the National Coalition for the Homeless.

[28] Austin, S. B., Ziyadeh, N. J., Corliss, H. L., Rosario, M., Wypij, D., Haines, J., Field, A. E. (2009). Sexual orientation disparities in purging and binge eating from early to late adolescence. The Journal of adolescent Health: Oficial Publication of the Society for Adolescent Medicine, 45(3), 238–245. doi:10.1016/j.jadohealth.2009.02.00

[29] Hu F. Measurements of Adiposity and Body Composition. In: Hu F, ed. Obesity Epidemiology. New York City: Oxford University Press, 2008; 53–83.

[30] Grodstein, F., Levine, R., Spencer, T., Colditz, G.A., & Stampfer, M.J. (1996). Three-year follow-up of participants in a commercial weight loss program. Can you keep it off? Archives of Internal Medicine, 156(12): 1302-6.

[31] Neumark-Sztainer, D., Wall, M., Guo, J., Story, M., Haines, J., & Eisenberg, M. (2006). Obesity, disordered eating, and eating disorders in a longitudinal study of adolescents: How

do dieters fare 5 years later? Journal of the American Dietetic Association, 106(4), 559-68.

32 Hudson, J.I, Hiripi, E., Pope, H.G., & Kessler, R. (2007). The prevalence and correlates of eating disorders in the national comorbidity survey replication. Biological Psychiatry, 61(3), 348-58.

33 Shisslak, C. M., Crago, M., & Estes, L. S. (1995). The spectrum of eating disturbances. International Journal of Eating Disorders, 18(3), 209-219.

34 Golden, N. H., Schneider, M., & Wood, C. (2016). Preventing obesity and eating disorders in adolescents. Pediatrics, 138(3). doi:10.1542/peds.2016-1649

35 Keys, A., Brozek, J., Henschel, A., Mickelsen, O., & Taylor, H.L. (1950). The biology of human starvation (2 volumes). Minneapolis, MN: University of Minnesota Press.

36 Maine, M., McGilley, H. & Burnell, D. (2010). Treatment of eating disorders: Bridging the gap. Academic Press: Maryland Heights, MO.

37 Frank, G. K., Shott, M. E., Riederer, J., & Pryor, T. L. (2016). Altered structural and effective connectivity in anorexia and bulimia nervosa in circuits that regulate energy and reward homeostasis. Translational Psychiatry, 6(11), e932. doi:10.1038/tp.2016.199

38 Bulik, C. (2014, December 1). Negative energy balance: A biological trap for people prone to anorexia nervosa. [Blog post]. Retrieved from https://uncexchanges.org/2014/12/01/negative-energy-balance-a-biological- trap-for-people-prone-to-anorexia-nervosa/.

[39] Goldield G.S., Adamo K.B., Rutherford J., Legg, C. (2008). Stress and the relative reinforcing value of food in female binge eaters. Physiology and Behavior, 93(3), 579–587.

[40] Van Oudenhove, L, McKie, S., Lassman, D., Uddin, B., Paine, P., Coen, S., Gregory, L., Tack, J., & Aziz, Q. (2011). Fatty acid–induced gut-brain signaling attenuates neural and behavioral effects of sad emotion in humans. The Journal of Clinical Investigation, 121(8), 3094-99.

[41] Wurtman, R., Wurtman, J., Regan, M., McDermott, J., Tsay, R., Breu, J. (2003). Effects of normal meals rich in carbohydrates or proteins on plasma tryptophan and tyrosine ratios. The American Journal of Clinical Nutrition. 77, 128-32.

[42] Epel, E.S., McEwen, B., Seeman, T., Matthews, K., Castellazzo, G., Brownell, K., Bell, J., Ickovics, J. (2000). Stress and body shape: stress-induced cortisol secretion is consistently greater among women with central fat. Psychosomatic Medicine. 62(5), 623-32.

[43] Lee, I., Shiroma, E.J., Kamada, M., Bassett, D.R., Matthews, C.E., Buring, J.E. (2019). Association of step volume and intensity with all-cause mortality in older women. JAMA Internal Medicine, 179(8), 1105-1112. doi: 10.1001/jamainternmed.2019.0899

[44] Pulsford, R.M., Stamatakis, E., Britton, A.R., Brunner, E.J., & Hillsdon, M. (2015). Associations of sitting behaviours with all-cause mortality over a 16- year follow-up: The Whitehall II study. International Journal of Epidemiology, 44(6), 1909–1916. https:/ doi.org/10.1093/ije/dyv191

[45] Van Uffelen, J.G.Z., Wong, J., Chau, J.Y., Van Der Ploeg, H.P., Riphagen, I., Gilson, N.D., Healy, G.N., Thorp, A.A., Clark, B.K., Gardiner, P.A., Dunstan, D.W., Bauman, A., Owen, N., & Brown, W.J. (2010). Occupational sitting and health risks. American Journal of Preventive Medicine, 39(4), 379-388.

46 Taheri, S., Lin, L., Austin, D., Young, T., & Mignot, E. (2004). Short sleep duration is associated with reduced leptin, elevated ghrelin, and increased body mass index (BMI). Sleep, 27, A146-A147. https:/ doi.org/10.1371/journal.pmed.0010062

47 Leproult, R., Copinsch,i G., Buxton, O., & Van Cauter, E. (1997). Sleep loss results in an elevation of cortisol levels the next evening. Sleep, 20, 865-870.

48 Ulfvebrand, S., Birgegard, A., Norring, C., Hogdahl, L., &Von Hausswolff- Juhlin, Y. (2015). Psychiatric comorbidity in women and men with eating disorders results from a large clinical database. Psychiatry Research, 230(2), 294-299.

49 Kaisari,P., Dourish, C.T., Rotshtein, P., & Higgs, S. (2018). Associations between core symptoms of attention deficit hyperactivity disorder and both binge and restrictive eating. Frontiers in Psychiatry, 9, 103. doi: 10.3389/fpsyt.2018.00103

Made in the USA
Columbia, SC
06 September 2020

19135417R00133